PUNCTUATION REVISITED

Punctuation Revisited is an advanced, comprehensive guide to the importance of punctuation in conveying meaning and augmenting the power of a message.

Richard Kallan provides guidance on how to structure sentences accurately and in a manner that enhances their readability and rhetorical appeal. This book discusses in fine detail not just when and how to employ specific punctuation marks, but the rationale behind them. The text also notes when the major academic style manuals differ in their punctuation advice. These unique features are designed to benefit beginning, intermediate, and advanced students of standard punctuation practice.

Punctuation Revisited is a wonderful resource for students of composition and writing, an essential read for writing center tutors and faculty, as well as the perfect addition to anyone's professional library.

Richard Kallan chairs the Communication Department at California State Polytechnic University, Pomona. He has taught writing at several colleges, including the University of Southern California (USC Marshall School of Business) and the University of California, Santa Barbara (Writing Program). Over the years, he has instructed courses spanning four disciplines: communication studies, journalism, English, and business.

PUNCTUATION REVISITED

A Strategic Guide for Academics, Wordsmiths, and Obsessive Perfectionists

[. ! ? , ; : ' ( ) – " " / ' ' …]

Richard Kallan

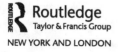
Routledge
Taylor & Francis Group

NEW YORK AND LONDON

First published 2020
by Routledge
52 Vanderbilt Avenue, New York, NY 10017

and by Routledge
2 Park Square, Milton Park, Abingdon, Oxon, OX14 4RN

Routledge is an imprint of the Taylor & Francis Group, an informa business

© 2020 Taylor & Francis

Library of Congress Cataloging-in-Publication Data
A catalog record for this title has been requested

ISBN: 978-1-138-33827-2 (hbk)
ISBN: 978-1-138-33828-9 (pbk)
ISBN: 978-0-429-44182-0 (ebk)

Typeset in Bembo
by Apex CoVantage, LLC

For my brother, Neal, and my sister, Linda.
Now, of course, you both owe *me* a dedication.

CONTENTS

ACKNOWLEDGMENTS

This book evolved and matured because of the astute recommendations of colleagues along the way. I am indebted to Darla Anderson, whose meticulous reading of multiple drafts of the manuscript led to a more accessible, audience-centered text; Olga Griswold, whose nuanced critique helped refine key portions of my counsel and commentary; Rebecca Mills, whose attention to detail enhanced the clarity of my message; and Micayla Anderson, who served as a research assistant and provided insightful perspective on the innovative uses of punctuation.

AUTHOR'S BACKGROUND

Richard Kallan chairs the Department of Communication at California State Polytechnic University, Pomona. He has taught writing at several colleges, including the University of Southern California (USC Marshall School of Business) and the University of California, Santa Barbara (Writing Program). Over the years, he has instructed courses spanning four disciplines: communication studies, journalism, English, and business.

Kallan is the author of *Renovating Your Writing: Shaping Ideas and Arguments into Clear, Concise, and Compelling Messages*, 2nd ed. (Routledge, 2018); *Armed Gunmen, True Facts, and Other Ridiculous Nonsense: A Compiled Compendium of Repetitive Redundancies* (Pantheon Books, 2005); and the coauthor of *How to Take the Fog Out of Business Writing* (Dartnell, 1994). He has also published scholarly articles in *Communication Monographs, Journalism & Mass Communication Quarterly, Journalism & Mass Communication Educator*, and *Journal of Popular Culture*.

INTRODUCTION

Punctuation refers to a set of marks or symbols that guide the reader in understanding the intended meaning of a sentence. These marks serve as cues for how to correctly read a sentence or, in other words, how to interpret what the writer is trying to say. English punctuation comprises fourteen marks: period, question mark, exclamation point, comma, semicolon, colon, dash, parentheses, brackets, apostrophe, double quotation marks, single quotation marks, ellipsis, and slash.[1]

As M. B. Parkes chronicles in *Pause and Effect: An Introduction to the History of Punctuation in the West*, punctuation developed out of necessity, becoming "an essential component of written language."[2]

> In Antiquity, the written word was regarded as a record of the spoken word, and texts were usually read aloud. But from the sixth century onwards attitudes to the written word changed: writing came to be regarded as conveying information directly to the mind through the eye.... The written medium developed as a separate manifestation of language with a status equivalent to, but independent of that of the spoken counterpart. New conventions, such as word separation, features of layout and punctuation, were developed to make it easier for readers to extract the information conveyed in the written medium, and over the centuries these were gradually augmented and refined. These conventions were first developed in the early Middle Ages for writing Latin.... Because many had to learn Latin as a foreign language, there was a need for conventions which made it easier to read.[3]

In an often cited example of the importance of punctuation in communicating meaning, a college professor asked students how they would punctuate this sentence: *Woman without her man is nothing.* Depending on the student's perspective, one of two readings resulted: *Woman—without her man—is nothing. Woman: without her, man is nothing.* Time after time, punctuation errors, such as the absence of a needed comma, may alter the writer's intended meaning. Sometimes the effect is comical, even to the point of inspiring the naming of a British pop band, *Let's Eat Grandma.* And although most punctuation errors do not affect the reader's understanding of the writer's intended meaning, such is not always the case. Omitting the Oxford comma (the last comma before the *and* in a series of items), in particular, can create confusion and misunderstanding. How, for example, might opposing attorneys interpret this statement: *My estate should be divided between Lucy, Harry and Riggs?* Does Lucy get one-half, or are all three entitled to equal shares of one-third?

Punctuation conveys meaning by suggesting how a sentence is meant to sound. Steven Pinker observes in *The Sense of Style: The Thinking Person's Guide to Writing in the 21st Century!*:

> In speech, the prosody of a sentence (its melody, rhythm, and pausing) eliminates any possibility of the hearer taking a wrong turn.... Punctuation, together with other graphical indicators such as italics, capitalization, and spacing, developed over the history of printed language ... provide the reader with hints about prosody, thus bringing writing a bit closer to speech.[4]

Some such as Wallace Chafe go so far as to argue that the primary function of punctuation is the "signaling of prosody" to help convey the sound of the writer's inner voice:

> Although punctuation certainly fails to represent the total range of prosodic phenomena a writer or reader may assign to a piece of written language, it does capture some major aspects of a writer's prosodic intent, to the extent that the quality and impact of a piece of writing may be greatly affected by the author's skill (or lack of it) in punctuating.[5]

Punctuation, of course, also imparts meaning by helping the reader navigate the syntax of a sentence. Beyond "restor[ing] some of the prosody ... that is missing from print," says Pinker, punctuation

> provides hints about the invisible syntactic tree that determines a sentence's meaning.... The problem for the writer is that punctuation indicates prosody in some places, syntax in others, and neither of them consistently anywhere. After centuries of chaos, the rules of punctuation began to settle down only a bit more than century ago, and even today the rules differ on the two sides of the Atlantic and from one publication to another.[6]

Punctuation differs from grammar, usage, and mechanics, although they are all commonly called *grammar,* a term popularly misappropriated to mean anything having to do with the "rules of writing." More accurately, **grammar** constitutes the rules governing a sentence's structural relationships, which include, for instance, how agreement is achieved between a sentence's various parts of speech. It is why we say *they* [subject] *are* [verb], not *they is.* **Usage** involves the correct use of a word or phrase, according to contemporary standards (for example, *affect* vs. *effect, imply* vs. *infer, uninterested* vs. *disinterested*). **Mechanics** encompasses the graphic conventions for dealing with technical matters specific to written language, such as how numbers are represented, how words are spelled and abbreviated, and what words are capitalized, italicized, and hyphenated.

Functions of Punctuation

Beyond helping the reader understand the meaning of a sentence, punctuation serves other key functions.

Punctuation elevates the coherence of your message by enhancing the structure of your thought. The very process of making punctuation decisions, especially when choices present themselves, compels you to closely examine how the elements of your sentence articulate with one another with respect to which are coordinate, subordinate, and superior. Punctuation thus allows you to capture and convey the hierarchy of your thoughts. As such, proficiency in punctuation becomes particularly helpful when writing longer, more complex sentences, whose effective structuring—and consequent readability and comprehension—requires appropriate punctuation. This is often the case in academic writing, where the complexity of thought and the need for layered and nuanced qualification lead to lengthy sentences; effective punctuation can significantly aid in the challenge of their processing.

Punctuation allows for a more powerful expression of your ideas. Curiously, this function of punctuation is seldom emphasized. From grade school on, punctuation lessons almost always focus on the *rules*, rather than the *power*, of punctuation. Yet, when used strategically, various marks—notably the colon, dash, semicolon, question mark, and ellipsis—can enhance, sometimes dramatically, the meaning and impact of your message. A well-placed colon, for example, enables you to make your point quickly and strikingly. *Asked whether she could ever be friends with someone who did not care about punctuation, her answer was unequivocal: no.* Even the modest period can powerfully advance an idea. As creatively illustrated in texting and tweeting—which ironically eschew many forms of punctuation—innovative practitioners have shown the power of the period to highlight key content by slowing down its processing. *I. will. not. do. your. homework. now. or. ever.* "Far from hindering creativity," as I noted in an earlier work, "knowing punctuation aids the process."[7]

Punctuation use/misuse characterizes your writing skills and, correspondingly, your perceived intelligence and competence. Yes, many punctuation errors go undetected by audiences, thereby never harming your credibility. But errors recognized by your reader are another matter. They can lower your credibility and the overall appeal of your message depending on how often they occur, how gross or comical the error, and what your audience expects of you (the audience for a text message, for example, is likely to be more forgiving of miscues than the audience for an academic paper). Conversely, a sophisticated use of punctuation will elevate your credibility with like-minded readers who value comprehensive writing skills. And because many of us have trouble with even the simplest of marks, a proficiency in punctuation distinguishes you from the crowd, increasing your worth to nearly any organization or employer.

To be sure, effective punctuation benefits all written messages from the least formal to the most formal. Moreover, the careful, nuanced application of punctuation fosters a mindset hallmarked by an attention to detail and perfection, which augments every aspect of your writing.

Why This Book?

But do we really need yet another punctuation lesson, let alone an entire book, devoted to the subject? No shortage of composition handbooks exists that treat—in addition to punctuation—grammar, usage, mechanics, and other topics. And scores of popular trade books on writing include sections on punctuation. Still, punctuation errors abound, many of us continually struggling to get it right. Even advanced writers—when they do make "rules-type" writing errors—seem to stumble more on punctuation than on grammar, usage, or mechanics. What is it about punctuation that makes it so challenging for so many?

This text is premised on the belief that punctuation instruction would make more sense and better resonate with readers if mentors were to (1) discuss in finer, more exacting detail when and how to employ each mark, (2) provide multiple examples of the mark used correctly and incorrectly, and (3) explain how choices in punctuation characterize the writer and impact the message. These features of the text are designed to benefit beginning, intermediate, and advanced students of *standard* punctuation practice.

The standard, however, remains fluid and evolving. "Perhaps that is why," David Crystal writes in *Making a Point: The Persnickety Story of English Punctuation*, "we care so much about punctuation: we are aware that its character is shifting and unpredictable, that it doesn't offer the same level of order and correctness that is seen in spelling and grammar, and it disturbs us."[8] And while Crystal argues for a more pragmatic approach to punctuation—by which he means "respecting all linguistic realities, whether rule-based or not"—he cautions:

> Being pragmatic doesn't mean "anything goes"—ignoring the rules that do exist.... The whole point of a standard language is to ensure general intelligibility and acceptability by having everyone follow an agreed and respected set of norms of usage.[9]

Even when one chooses to depart from those norms, the reader benefits when the writer's decision-making is informed by a mastery of standard practice.

Organization of Chapters

Each chapter offers an extended discussion of the mark's purpose and application, beginning with the basic, most common uses of the mark before proceeding to those less typically encountered situations, found mainly in academic and scholarly writing, calling for the mark's use and specific positioning. The guidelines illustrate how to punctuate sentence structures ranging from the simplest to the most complex. Each chapter also describes how the mark can rhetorically depict the writer and his/her text.

Chapter 1 covers the three easiest marks to learn: the period, question mark, and exclamation point. These marks indicate when a sentence (or incomplete sentence) has ended and whether it is declaring, asking, or exclaiming.

Chapter 2, on the other hand, explores the most difficult mark to master, the comma, which is used to separate words or word groupings as they appear in a variety of sentence structures. Many comma decisions are devoid of debate or controversy. Other times, whether a comma is needed is not so readily apparent, even when one knows the principles governing its use.

Chapter 3 expounds on semicolons, which connect related ideas, usually in the form of independent clauses; or they provide greater, needed separation of items or ideas within a complex series of items or ideas.

Chapter 4 focuses on colons and dashes, marks that primarily introduce, highlight, or expand upon items or ideas.

Chapter 5 provides a tutorial on how apostrophes signal possession, create contractions, and form certain plurals.

Chapter 6 addresses double quotation marks and single quotation marks, whose primary function is to acknowledge the words of another, in addition to indicating titles of works and calling attention to certain words.

Chapter 7 shows how ellipses and slashes signal that something has been left out of the sentence to save space and move the reader more quickly to your point. The chapter also demonstrates how quoted material can be editorially synthesized.

Chapter 8 discusses parentheses and brackets, which serve to structurally subordinate information.

It is important to recognize that punctuation marks function neither discretely nor distinctively from one another; rather, the use of any one mark often intersects with another. Knowing how to use quotation marks, for example, entails also knowing about commas, ellipses, parentheses, and brackets, as well as knowing where to place periods, question marks, and exclamation points. A strictly linear discussion of punctuation is impossible, despite the organizational efforts reflected in the chapter summaries above. Out of necessity, the discussion of punctuation presented is sometimes recursive.

Although the most prominent academic style manuals—notably *The Chicago Manual of Style*,[10] *MLA Handbook for Writers of Research Papers*,[11] and the *Publication Manual of the American Psychological Association*[12]—generally agree on the basic conventions of punctuation, they sometimes differ on when to use and/or how to position certain marks; these variances, when relevant, will be identified throughout the text. The more frequent and significant differences that occur between academic style manuals and *The Associated Press Stylebook and Briefing on Media Law*,[13] which informs the punctuation practices of most newspapers and many popular periodicals, will similarly be referenced. Key distinctions between British usage of certain marks, as delineated in the *New Oxford Style Manual*,[14] and American usage of those marks will be explained as well.

Finally, some cautionary comments:

No book about punctuation, however detailed, can anticipate and address every issue that may arise from the unique content of a specific text. Faced with ambiguous, let alone sometimes conflicting, guidelines, the writer must choose sensibly and consistently. A thorough and keen understanding of the logic of punctuation facilitates that process.

Occasionally, the correct use of punctuation in certain instances can result in an odd-looking and/or awkward-sounding sentence (*My friend's aunt's next-door neighbor's dog ...*) that is more difficult to process than if it were rewritten (*The dog belonging to the next-door neighbor of my friend's aunt ...*). Structurally recasting a sentence to eliminate cumbersome punctuation is always an option.

Quality writing is much more than the mastery of punctuation. Sometimes in the haste of meeting a deadline or in the process of experimenting stylistically, even accomplished writers commit punctuation errors. It happens, the world does not end, and—spoiler alert—life goes on. Confident writers know that it is better to risk making a mistake than to obsess about correctness, forever playing it safe and continually steering clear of the kind of stylistic invention and creativity that gives writing its personality and character.

I would be remiss if I did not acknowledge having refrained at times from including the kind of detail about various marks that seemed so arcane (i.e., even more arcane than the material I did choose to include!), or so unique to a particular sentence structure, it might be more distracting than informative. The goal was to produce a thorough and precise punctuation guide that was still practical, accessible, and reader-friendly.

Notes

1 Not included in this list are braces, bullets, en dashes, and hyphens, which, while sometimes referred to as punctuation, speak more to graphic design and mechanics. Chapter 3, however, does discuss how to punctuate the text that follows a bullet, and Chapter 4 shows how a colon introduces a bulleted list.

2 M.B. Parkes, *Pause and Effect: An Introduction to the History of Punctuation in the West* (Berkeley: University of California Press, 1993), 1.

3 Parkes, *Pause and Effect*, 1.
4 Steven Pinker, *The Sense of Style: The Thinking Person's Guide to Writing in the 21st Century!* (New York: Viking, 2014), 120–21.
5 William Chafe, "Punctuation and the Prosody of Written Language," in *Landmark Essays on Speech and Writing*, ed. Peter Elbow (New York: Routledge, 2015), 202.
6 Pinker, *The Sense of Style*, 284.
7 Richard Kallan, *Renovating Your Writing: Shaping Ideas and Arguments into Clear, Concise, and Compelling Messages*, 2nd ed. (New York: Routledge, 2018), 172–73.
8 David Crystal, *Making a Point: The Persnickety Story of English Punctuation* (New York: St. Martin's Press, 2015), 344.
9 Crystal, *Making a Point*, 345, 347–48.
10 University of Chicago Press, *The Chicago Manual of Style*, 17th ed. (Chicago: University of Chicago Press, 2017). Hereafter referenced as *Chicago*.
11 The Modern Language Association of America, *MLA Handbook for Writers of Research Papers*, 7th ed. (New York: The Modern Language Association of America, 2009). The 7th edition includes an extended discussion of punctuation; the latest edition—The Modern Language Association of America, *MLA Handbook*, 8th ed. (New York: The Modern Language Association of America, 2016)—does not. Hereafter referenced as *MLA*, 7th ed. or *MLA*, 8th ed.
12 American Psychological Association, *Publication Manual of the American Psychological Association*, 6th ed. (Washington, DC: American Psychological Association, 2010). Hereafter referenced as *APA*.
13 The Associated Press, *The Associated Press Stylebook 2018 and Briefing on Media Law* (New York: The Associated Press, 2018). Hereafter referenced as *AP Stylebook*.
14 *New Oxford Style Manual* (Oxford: Oxford University Press, 2016). Hereafter referenced as *Oxford Style*.

1

PERIODS, QUESTION MARKS, AND EXCLAMATION POINTS

Purpose and Application

Commonly referred to as "ending punctuation," periods, question marks, and exclamation points can be placed *almost* anywhere. They usually come at the end of a complete sentence, but they can also follow an incomplete sentence, whether in the form of a dependent clause, phrase, or single word. These marks indicate when a sentence (or incomplete sentence) has ended and whether it is declaring, asking, or exclaiming. More challenging is the correct positioning of periods, question marks, and exclamation points when they are used in conjunction with other forms of punctuation.

QUICK REFERENCE GLOSSARY

A **COMPLETE SENTENCE** features one or more independent clauses. An **independent clause** is a related word grouping that can stand alone as a sentence because it (1) includes a subject and a predicate and (2) expresses a complete thought.

1. The **subject** is who or what initiates or receives whatever is happening in the sentence. The **predicate** describes the happening; it commences with a **verb**, which most often is an action, and usually comprises one or more other elements (a direct object, an indirect object, a complement, and modifiers).

> I [subject] enjoy [verb] my writing class.
> I [subject] enjoy my writing class [predicate].

Other times, the verb establishes a *condition* by serving as a **linking verb** that, in essence, functions much like an equal sign to connect the subject and the condition.

> Writing is fun.
> Writing = fun.
> Writing [subject] is [linking verb] fun [condition].
> Writing [subject] is fun [predicate].

Sometimes the subject of a sentence is implied, such as a command.

> Run [predicate]!

The implied subject of any command where the subject is **not** explicitly stated is always *you*.

2. Along with having a subject and a predicate, a complete sentence expresses a **complete thought**: a "finished" declaration, exclamation/command, or question. Note how these sentences have a subject and a predicate but remain incomplete:

> Although I love to write.
> When class starts.
> If I may ask.

Each sentence is incomplete because the writer begins but never finishes the larger thought the sentence structure promises. Instead, we have three dependent (or subordinate) clauses. A **dependent** (or **subordinate**) **clause** contains a subject and a predicate, but it does **not** express a complete thought. Unable to stand alone, a dependent clause must precede or follow an independent clause to form a complete sentence. Dependent clauses are introduced with **subordinating conjunctions**, such as *after, although, as, because, before, even if, even though, if, since, so that, than, that, though, unless, until, when, whenever, where, whereas, wherever, whether, while.*

An INCOMPLETE SENTENCE (also referred to as a **sentence fragment**) takes the form of either a dependent clause; a **phrase**, which is a related word grouping that does **not** have both a subject and a predicate; or a single (non-command) word. *Because those are the rules. All right readers, any questions? Good.*

Adapted from Richard Kallan, *Renovating Your Writing: Shaping Ideas and Arguments into Clear, Concise, and Compelling Messages.* 2nd ed., Routledge, 2018. Permission courtesy of Routledge.

Periods

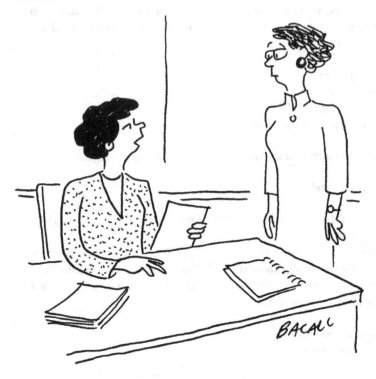

"I think I use the Internet too much. I find myself writing 'com' after each period."

Bacall, Aaron; www.CartoonStock.com

Ending a Sentence

1.1 The most common use of a period is to end a sentence. Like the question mark and the exclamation point, it tells the reader to stop.

Leave one space after a period. Just like at the start of this sentence. **Not** like the start of this one. The standard now is to leave *one* space after all punctuation, including periods, question marks, exclamation points, and colons.

- This is an example of a sentence that ends with a period.
- This is another example. And here's one more.

Most sentences end with periods. If a sentence does **not** end with a period, it will likely end with a question mark or an exclamation point. The exceptions would be a sentence ending in "suspension points," a name given to a specific use of ellipsis, which is formatted with **no** ending punctuation (see Chapter 7: 7.12); or a sentence ending in a dash used to signal interrupted speech (see Chapter 4: 4.22).

Providing Visual Closure

1.2 Periods provide *visual closure* at the end of incomplete sentences, stopping them from flowing into the sentences (and incomplete sentences) that follow. Periods also provide visual closure when phrases and single words serve as in-text headings; the period separates the heading from the text.

> I am qualified to become your social media director for three reasons:
>> TECHNICAL SKILLS. I am proficient in …
>> WORK EXPERIENCE. My industry experience includes working at …
>> EDUCATION BACKGROUND. As my resume details, I earned a BA from …

Do **not**, however, place periods after article and essay titles, chapter titles, headings and subheadings (even if they form complete sentences), and captions for photographs and illustrations that are incomplete sentences. (Periods, though, should follow multiple sentences, incomplete sentences, or a combination of both when they comprise a caption.)

Following Abbreviations[1]

1.3 Place periods after abbreviations of titles.

> Col. Dr. Gen. Hon. Messrs. Mr. Mrs. Ms. Rev.

1.4 The trend is away from using periods with academic degrees. Nearly all major style manuals recommend such, with the exception of *AP Stylebook*. The preferred style (with some exceptions—LL.M, LL.D):

> AA BA BS BFA MA MS MFA MBA
> PhD PsyD EdD MD RN JD

1.5 Place periods after abbreviations common to informal (and sometimes formal) writing.

> a.m.   apt.   ave.   etc.   p.m.   p.s.   oz.
> lbs.   inc.   jr.   sr.   Jan. (and other months)

Note: No space comes between the letters of a two-word abbreviation: a.m. (**not** a. m.).

1.6 Place periods after abbreviations often found in academic citations.

> ch.   ed.   e.g.   et al.   i.e.   no.   nos.
> p.   pp.   rev.   sect.   trans.   vol.   vols.

1.7 Style manuals sometimes differ as to whether *initialisms*, abbreviations created by combining the first capitalized letter of each word in a name or phrase, require periods. Most often, the periods are dropped.

> AD   BC   CEO   CIA   CD   CNN   DNA   ESL
> FBI   LGBT   LGBTQIA   MBA   MIT   MVP   NAACP
> NBA   NBC   NFL   RSVP   UCLA   US   USA

Acronyms, which are essentially initialisms pronounced as words, **not** as individualized initials, follow the same pattern.

> AIDS   ASAP   AWOL   ICE   MADD   MASH   NAFTA   NASA
> NATO   OPEC   PETA   (Navy) SEALS   SWAT   UNICEF

No spaces come between the letters comprising an initialism or acronym.

1.8 Place a period followed by a space after each initial comprising part of a name.

> F. Scott Fitzgerald   Hunter S. Thompson   J. K. Rowling   J. R. R. Tolkien

But when a name comprises only initials, **no** period or space follows each initial.

> FDR   JFK   LBJ   MLK

1.9 Do **not** place periods after postal abbreviations, compass points, or time zones.

> AL   CA   MA   NY   OH   PA   TX
> N   S   E   W   NE   NW   SE   SW
> EST   CDT   MST   PDT

1.10 When a sentence concludes with an abbreviation ending in a period, the period also ends the sentence; **no** additional period is needed.

- I love all forms of punctuation: periods, question marks, exclamation points, commas, semicolons, etc.
- My English teacher said that I "end too many sentences with *etc.*"
- She gave me a book, *Two Words to Avoid in Formal Writing: Etc. and Misc.* I stayed up reading it until 1:30 a.m.

Following Numbered and Lettered Items

1.11 Place periods, without parentheses, after vertically formatted numbers and letters that come before lists. Like this:

  1. text ...   A. text ...
  2. text ...   B. text ...
  3. text ...   C. text ...

Not like this:

  (1) text ...   (A) text ...
  (2) text ...   (B) text ...
  (3) text ...   (C) text ...

  (1.) text ...   (A.) text ...
  (2.) text ...   (B.) text ...
  (3.) text ...   (C.) text ...

  1) text ...   A) text ...
  2) text ...   B) text ...
  3) text ...   C) text ...

  1.) text ...   A.) text ...
  2.) text ...   B.) text ...
  3.) text ...   C.) text ...

It is **not** necessary to place parentheses around vertically formatted numbers or letters because the period alone sufficiently separates the number/letter visually from the text that follows. On the other hand, *in-text* numbering and lettering must be enclosed in parentheses (double, **not** single) to effectively separate the numbering and lettering from the subsequent text. Like this:

- Three steps must be taken: (1) text ... (2) text ... (3) text ...
- Three steps must be taken: (A) text ... (B) text ... (C) text ...

Not like this, where the periods are unnecessary:

- Three steps must be taken: (1.) text … (2.) text … (3.) text …
- Three steps must be taken: (A.) text … (B.) text … (C.) text …

Parentheses should be paired (see Chapter 8: 8.4), like this:

- Three steps must be taken: (1) text … (2) text … (3) text …
- Three steps must be taken: (A) text … (B) text … (C) text …

Not like this:

- Three steps must be taken: 1) text … 2) text … 3) text …
- Three steps must be taken: A) text … B) text … C) text …

Positioning with Quotation Marks and Italicized Titles

1.12 When a sentence ends with quoted material, the period goes inside the closing quotation mark, even if just one word is quoted.

- In *Woe Is I: The Grammarphobe's Guide to Better English in Plain English*, Patricia T. O'Conner says, "Think of quotation marks as bookends that support a quotation in between."[2]
- Jason followed every rule even though, he complained, it sometimes looked "weird."

1.13 If, however, a sentence ends with a word or phrase customarily placed in *single* quotation marks, a convention followed by some disciplines where certain words have specialized meanings (see Chapter 6: 6.21), the period comes after the second, single quotation mark but before the second, double quotation mark.

- Punctuation is my 'deity'.
- Lauren declared, "Punctuation is my 'deity'."

If 'deity' were to come at the end of an italicized title, the period would come last.

> Lauren authored a play, *Punctuation Is My 'Deity'*. [The period is **not** italicized.]

1.14 When a sentence ends with quoted material within quoted material, the period goes inside, or before, the closing, single quotation mark, unless it is proceeded by another quotation in double quotation marks.

- He wrote, "I read a fabulous article, 'Transcendental Punctuation.'"
- She wrote, "I read an intriguing article, 'Transcendental Grammar: Some Say, "No way."'"

Note: To enhance legibility, include a slight space between single and double quotation marks when positioned together: (' "), rather than ('").

Positioning with Parentheses

1.15 A period goes outside or inside a closing parenthesis, depending on the nature of the parenthetical material, as further explained and illustrated by the sentences below.

- A period goes outside the closing parenthesis when the sentence ends with an incomplete parenthetical sentence (such as a dependent clause, phrase, or word).
- A period goes outside the closing parenthesis when the sentence ends with a complete parenthetical sentence, i.e., an independent clause, which usually is neither capitalized nor followed with a period (this is an example).
- A period goes inside the closing parenthesis when a complete parenthetical sentence stands alone. (This is an example.)

1.16 **No** period follows a complete parenthetical sentence (this is an example) coming in the middle of a sentence; nor is the parenthetical sentence usually capitalized. However, in some cases, notably when referencing certain quotations, it is appropriate to capitalize a parenthetical sentence appearing within the sentence.

> The Declaration of Independence describes the essence of American thinking ("We hold these truths to be self-evident, that all men are created equal, that they are endowed by their Creator with certain unalienable Rights, that among these are Life, Liberty and the pursuit of Happiness") both past and present.

1.17 **No** period follows an incomplete parenthetical sentence, such as a dependent clause (when you write one), phrase (such as this), or (single) word coming in the middle of the sentence unless the parenthetical comment ends with an abbreviation (such as etc.). Nor is the clause, phrase, or word usually capitalized. On the other hand, question marks and exclamation points *do* follow complete and incomplete parenthetical sentences in the form of questions and exclamations (see 1.28 and 1.38).

Positioning with Footnotes/Endnotes

1.18 When footnotes/endnotes (superscripted numbers) are used, they usually follow the sentence's ending period (or other ending punctuation).

- I shared with classmates one of my favorite books, *Perfect Punctuation in an Imperfect World*.[fn]
- The author provides a great example of the importance of punctuation.[fn]
- I shared with classmates one of my favorite articles, "Punctuation Is Fun."[fn]
- He wrote, "I read a fabulous article, 'Transcendental Punctuation.'" [fn] [The note or in-text citation would reference where he wrote, "I read a fabulous article," and not necessarily where the article appeared; the same holds for the example below.]
- She wrote, "I read an intriguing article, 'Transcendental Grammar: Some Say, "No way."'"[fn]

Positioning with Parenthetical Information

1.19 When parenthetical information, such as an in-text citation, comes after a declarative sentence ending in quoted material, most style manuals recommend placing the period after the parenthesis. The same holds true when the parenthetical information comes after an italicized title or paraphrased text. (The in-text citation examples that follow conform to *Chicago* style, which lists the last name of the author(s) and then the date of publication, followed by the page number if the reference is to a specific passage; other style manuals, such *MLA*, do **not** include the date of publication in in-text citations.)

- I shared with classmates one of my favorite books, *Perfect Punctuation in an Imperfect World* (Perez 2019).
- The author provides a great example of the importance of punctuation (Perez 2019, 22–25).
- I shared with classmates one of my favorite articles, "Punctuation Is Fun" (James 2018).
- He wrote, "I read a fabulous article, 'Transcendental Punctuation'" (Goodwin 2017, 10).
- She wrote, "I read an intriguing article, 'Transcendental Grammar: Some Say, "No way"'" (Rowe 2019, 11).

1.20 When parenthetical information, such as an in-text citation, comes after a sentence that concludes with quoted material ending in a question mark or exclamation point, the period after the parenthesis is still maintained. The same holds true if the parenthetical information comes after an italicized title ending in a question mark or exclamation point.

- We listened to a speech, "Why Doesn't Everyone Love Punctuation?" (Barnett 2017).
- The writer proclaimed, "I adore punctuation!" (Fong 2017, 3).
- My therapist bought me a three volume self-help series, *Can Proper Punctuation Benefit Your Marriage?* (Johnson 2016).
- This new collection of poetry caught my attention: *The Poetry of Punctuation!* (Kang 2019).

Question Marks

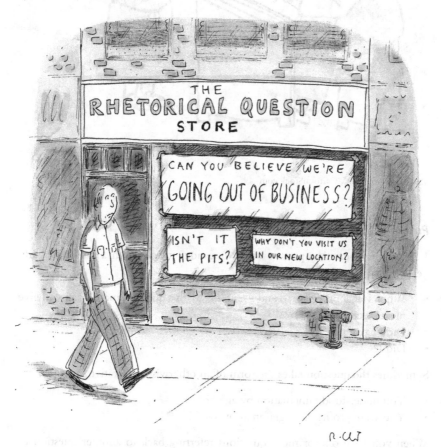

Roz Chast/The New Yorker Collection/The Cartoon Bank; Condé Nast

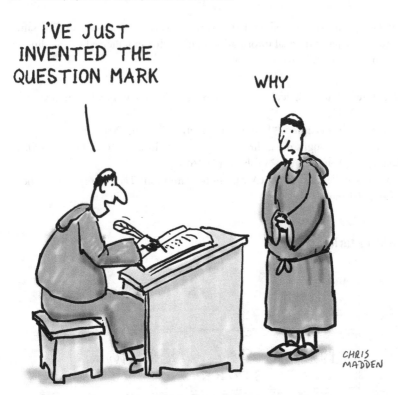

Madden, Chris; www.CartoonStock.com

Posing a Direct Question

1.21 When a sentence poses a direct question, it ends with a question mark. Leave one space after a question mark.

- When is it appropriate to end a sentence with a question mark? Can you give me an example?
- Didn't you just give me two?
- Did I?

Sometimes the question takes the form of an otherwise declarative sentence.

- You understood punctuation by age 5?
- You were proficient at grammar by age 7?

When you have one or more questions referring back to another question or another sentence, punctuate them with question marks even if they are **not** complete sentences.

Where did you learn how to use a question mark so effectively? In junior high? High school? College? Or was it when you dated that Philosophy major?

Posing an Indirect Question

1.22 Do **not** use a question mark (or quotation marks) when posing an indirect question. An indirect question paraphrases your own question or someone else's question in such a way that it is no longer a direct inquiry.

- I asked my teacher if she enjoyed teaching punctuation.
- I cannot decide whether I am using too many question marks or whether I am not using enough.
- My professors want to know why I care so much about punctuation and why I just don't focus on writing clearly, concisely, and compellingly.
- Their friends wondered whether such opposites—a punctuation lover and punctuation hater—would remain a couple.

Following Abbreviations

1.23 When you, the writer, pose a question that concludes with an abbreviation ending in a period, the question mark comes after the period. Should parenthetical information follow the abbreviation, the question mark comes after the closing parenthesis.

- Are you aware of the latest research on practicing punctuation at 5 a.m.?
  Are you aware of the latest research on practicing punctuation at 5 a.m. (Kim 2019)?
- When will we discuss "Practicing Punctuation at 5 A.M."?
  When will we discuss "Practicing Punctuation at 5 A.M." (Kim 2019)?
- When will we discuss *Mastering Grammar at 5 A.M.*?
  When will we discuss *Mastering Grammar at 5 A.M.* (Washington 2018)?

Positioning with Quotation Marks and Italicized Titles

1.24 When a sentence concludes with quoted material ending in a question mark, the mark goes *inside* the closing double quotation mark (or, occasionally, *inside* a closing single quotation mark should one follow a double quotation mark). The question mark serves as ending punctuation; **no** subsequent period is needed.

- We read a wonderful essay, "Does Everyone—and I Mean *Everyone*— Overuse the Dash?"

- She asked, "Is the dash really overused, especially by those her Journalism teacher dismissed as 'second-thought writers'?"
- She asked, "Is the dash really overused, especially by those her Journalism teacher dismissed as 'second-thought writers with names like "Ace"?'"

1.25 When a sentence concludes with an italicized title ending in a question mark, the (italicized) question mark serves as ending punctuation; **no** subsequent period is needed.

> I started a new blog, *So You Think You Can Punctuate?*

1.26 When a sentence concludes with quoted material or an italicized title **not** ending in a question mark, but you, the writer, are posing a question, the question mark goes *outside* the closing quotation mark or at the end of the italicized title.

- Did you like the short story, "The Prince and Princess of Punctuation"?
- Did you like the graphic novel, *Epic Battle over the Oxford Comma*? [The question mark is **not** italicized.]
- Have you seen Goodwin's Facebook post, "I read a fabulous article, 'Transcendental Punctuation'"?
- Have you seen Rowe's Facebook post, "I read an intriguing article, 'Transcendental Grammar: Some Say, "No way"'"?

1.27 When you, the writer, are posing a question, and parenthetical information (such as an in-text citation) follows the quoted material or italicized title, most style manuals recommend placing the question mark after the closing parenthesis.

- Did you like the short story, "The Prince and Princess of Punctuation" (Riggs 2019)?
- Did you like the graphic novel, *Epic Battle over the Oxford Comma* (Harry 2019)?

Positioning with Parentheses

1.28 When a parenthetical question in the form of a complete sentence comes in the middle of another sentence (do you see what I mean?) or at the end of a sentence, a question mark follows the parenthetical question (that make sense, right?). Generally, the question is **not** capitalized; below is an exception.

> In my interview for Director of the Punctuation Institute, one question (What advice would you give a writer when confronting a sentence structure where either a colon or a dash seems appropriate?) proved especially difficult.

1.29 An incomplete parenthetical sentence ending in a question mark is **not** capitalized.

> She said she loved dependent clauses (as if anyone didn't?), phrases (any old phrase?), and words (really?).

Positioning with Other Forms of Punctuation

1.30 When a sentence concludes with quoted material or an italicized title ending in a question mark and you, the writer, are also posing a question, one question mark suffices.

- Why haven't you referenced "Can Mastery of the Semicolon Change Your Life?"
  Why haven't you referenced "Can Mastery of the Semicolon Change Your Life?" (Neumann 2017).
- Why haven't you referenced *Should Toddlers Know How to Use an Ellipsis?*
  Why haven't you referenced *Should Toddlers Know How to Use an Ellipsis?* (Bradley 2017).

1.31 When a sentence concludes with quoted material or an italicized title ending in an exclamation point and you, the writer, are posing a question, the long-standing convention had been for the exclamation point to take precedence and end the sentence; **no** question mark was added.

- Has anyone read "Punctuation Must Be Taught in Kindergarten!"
  Has anyone read "Punctuation Must Be Taught in Kindergarten!" (Mahoney 2018).
- Has anyone read *Grammar Must Be Taught in Kindergarten!*
  Has anyone read *Grammar Must Be Taught in Kindergarten!* (Dempsey 2019).

Chicago now advises, however, to add the question mark.[3]

- Has anyone read "Punctuation Must Be Taught in Kindergarten!"?
  Has anyone read "Punctuation Must Be Taught in Kindergarten!" (Mahoney 2018)?
- Has anyone read *Grammar Must Be Taught in Kindergarten!*? [The question mark is **not** italicized.]
  Has anyone read *Grammar Must Be Taught in Kindergarten!* (Dempsey 2019)?

This new guideline also applies when you, the writer, exclaim about quoted or italicized material ending in a question mark (see 1.41).

Exclamation Points

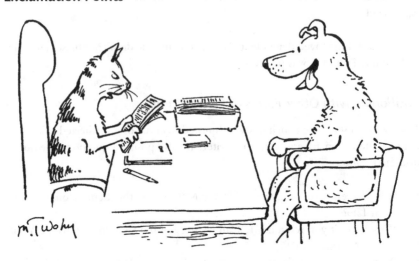

"You tend to overuse the exclamation point."

Mike Twohy/The New Yorker Collection/The Cartoon Bank; Condé Nast

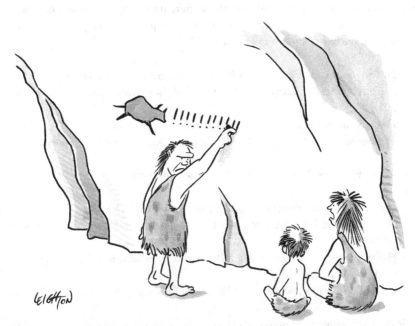

"O.K., we get it—big and dangerous."

Robert Leighton/The New Yorker Collection/The Cartoon Bank; Condé Nast

Following Exclamations

1.32 When a sentence or incomplete sentence exclaims, it ends with an exclamation point, which is usually positioned at the end of the sentence. Leave one space after an exclamation point.

- I love exclamation points! They're awesome! They're amazing! Just marvelous!
- Stop it! You're using too many exclamation points!
- No! Don't tell me what to do! Ever again!

Following Abbreviations

1.33 When you, the writer, exclaim and the sentence concludes with an abbreviation ending in a period, the exclamation point follows the period. Should parenthetical information follow the abbreviation, the exclamation point comes after the parenthesis.

- You must become aware of the recent research on practicing punctuation at 5 a.m.!
  You must become aware of the recent research on practicing punctuation at 5 a.m. (Kim 2019)!
- You must read "Practicing Punctuation at 5 A.M."!
  You must read "Practicing Punctuation at 5 A.M." (Kim 2019)!
- You must read *Mastering Grammar at 5 A.M.*!
  You must read *Mastering Grammar at 5 A.M.* (Washington 2018)!

Positioning with Quotation Marks and Italicized Titles

1.34 The positioning of an exclamation point with quoted material follows the same logic guiding the question mark. When a sentence concludes with quoted material ending in an exclamation point, the point goes *inside* the closing double quotation mark (or, occasionally, *inside* a closing single quotation mark should one follow a double quotation mark). The exclamation point serves as ending punctuation; **no** subsequent period is needed.

- Assigned readings included "Punctuation Must Be Taught in Kindergarten!"
- Her journalism teacher loudly exclaimed, "The dash is overused, especially by those I have called 'second-thought writers'!"
- Her journalism teacher loudly exclaimed, "The dash is overused, especially by those I have called 'second-thought writers with names like "Ace"'!"

1.35 When a sentence concludes with an italicized title ending in an exclamation point, the italicized exclamation point serves as ending punctuation; **no** subsequent period is needed.

> Assigned readings included *Grammar Must Be Taught in Kindergarten!*

1.36 When a sentence concludes with quoted material or an italicized title **not** ending in anexclamation point, but you, the writer, are exclaiming, the exclamation point goes *outside* the closing quotation mark or at the end of the italicized title.

- Drop everything immediately and read the short story, "The Prince and Princess of Punctuation"!
- Drop everything immediately and read the graphic novel, *Epic Battle over the Oxford Comma*! [The exclamation point is **not** italicized.]
- You must immediately check out Goodwin's Facebook post, "I read a fabulous article, 'Transcendental Punctuation'"!
- You must immediately check out Rowe's Facebook post, "I read an intriguing article, 'Transcendental Grammar: Some Say, "No way"'"!

1.37 When you, the writer, are exclaiming, and parenthetical information (such as an in-text citation) follows the quoted material or italicized title, most style manuals recommend placing the exclamation point after the parenthesis.

- Drop everything immediately and read "The Prince and Princess of Punctuation" (Riggs 2019)!
- Drop everything immediately and read the graphic novel, *Epic Battle over the Oxford Comma* (Harry 2019)!

Positioning with Parentheses

1.38 When a parenthetical exclamation in the form of a complete sentence, i.e., an independent clause, comes in the middle of a sentence (this is a terrific example!) or at the end of the sentence, the parenthetical exclamation ends with an exclamation point, but it generally—see exception below—is **not** capitalized (these distinctions are so much fun!).

> His membership in the Pomona Punctuation Club was revoked because he continually violated one of its most sacred guiding rules governing exclamation points (Thou shall not use exclamation marks indiscriminately!).

1.39 An incomplete parenthetical sentence ending in an exclamation point is **not** capitalized. This holds true for a parenthetical exclamation appearing as a dependent clause (which I will now illustrate!), phrase (regardless of whether short or long!), or word (yes!).

Positioning with Other Forms of Punctuation

1.40 When a sentence concludes with quoted material or an italicized title ending in an exclamation point and you, the writer, are also exclaiming, one exclamation point suffices.

- Drop everything immediately and read "Punctuation Must Be Taught in Kindergarten!"
  Drop everything immediately and read "Punctuation Must Be Taught in Kindergarten!" (Mahoney 2018).
- Drop everything immediately and read *Grammar Must Be Taught in Kindergarten!*
  Drop everything immediately and read *Grammar Must Be Taught in Kindergarten!* (Dempsey 2019).

1.41 When a sentence concludes with quoted material or an italicized title ending in a question mark and you, the writer, are exclaiming, the long-standing convention (similar to that of posing a question at the end of an exclamation—see 1.31) had been for the question mark to take precedence and end the sentence; **no** exclamation point was added. *Chicago* now advises, however, to add the exclamation point.[4]

- Drop everything immediately and read "Can Mastery of the Semicolon Change Your Life?"!
  Drop everything immediately and read "Can Mastery of the Semicolon Change Your Life?" (Neumann 2017)!
- Drop everything immediately and read *Should Toddlers Know How to Use an Ellipsis?*! [The exclamation point is **not** italicized.]
  Drop everything immediately and read *Should Toddlers Know How to Use an Ellipsis?* (Bradley 2017)!

RHETORICALLY SPEAKING

Periods

The short sentence (or phrase or word) abruptly ending in a period can powerfully drive home your point.

- The school's policy on campus skateboarding was seldom observed. But no one seemed to care. Not the teachers. Not the students. Nobody.
- Would the policy ever be changed? No.

As illustrated under "Providing Visual Closure" (see 1.2), a period following a phrase or word corrals and highlights the text, momentarily stopping the reader.

In highly informal writing, such as texting and tweeting, the period has been creatively used to emphasize key content by slowing down its processing. *I. never. cheated. ever.* Sometimes the absence of periods (and all other punctuation) tries to convey the writer's out-of-breath excitement. *I saw a new band on Saturday they were great I mean really fabulous I absolutely loved them I know you will love them let's go see them next week.*

More commonplace, however, is the omission of periods in highly informal writing. "One of the cardinal rules of texting," Jeff Guo reminds us, "is that you *don't use periods, period.* Not unless you want to come off as cold, angry or passive-aggressive.... The period ... has become the evil twin of the exclamation point. It's now an optional mark that adds emphasis—but a nasty, dour sort of emphasis."[5] Moreover, Danielle Gunraj discovered that "text messages that ended with a period were rated as less sincere than text messages that did not end with a period. This pattern, however, was not found for handwritten notes."[6] Concludes David Crystal: "In an instant message, it is pretty obvious a sentence has come to an end, and none will have a full stop. So why use it."[7]

These innovative uses—and non-uses—of punctuation, it should be stressed, are appropriate and acceptable in specific, limited venues, which do not yet include many traditional, more formal writing contexts.

Question Marks

The rhetorical question (a question to which you already know the answer) can dramatically express your point.

> The candidate's application letter to be senior editor contained three grammatical errors, four punctuation mistakes, and five instances of odd usage. Is this who we want editing our corporate publications?

The allure of the rhetorical question and its ease of application, however, often results in its overuse.

> She claims that punctuation is overrated. Overrated? Is she on drugs? Or just acting like she's drugged out? And she calls herself a serious student? Really? I mean, really? Do you think we should tell her parents? Why not?

Richly expressive, the question mark can even stand alone, functioning not as ending punctuation but as editorial commentary that signals the writer's doubt.

> He claimed that the best diet food was pizza (?), and that within the last two months he had lost 200 pounds (??) eating pizza every day.

Exclamation Points

Similar to question marks, exclamation points should be used sparingly in formal writing, their overuse suggesting an unseasoned writer who lacks the tools to express passion and intensity in more sophisticated ways.

Even occasional use of exclamation points may be frowned upon. Academics, in particular, customarily let their scholarship speak for itself, without resorting to announcements of the material's importance. Rarely do exclamation points appear in scholarly writing.

The exclamation point is also eschewed by novelists. F. Scott Fitzgerald famously said, "An exclamation point is like laughing at your own joke,"[8] while Elmore Leonard declares, "You are allowed no more than two or three per 100,000 words of prose," although he grants, "If you have the knack of playing with exclaimers the way Tom Wolfe does, you can throw them in by the handful."[9] Most novelists only occasionally use exclamation points.

On the other hand, the exclamation point can convey friendliness and support for the reader. Carol Waseleski, in her study of "Gender and the Use of Exclamation Points in Computer-Mediated Communication: An Analysis of Exclamations Posted to Two Electronic Discussion Lists," confirms that while women use exclamation points more than men, the points do not "function solely—or even very often—as markers of excitability." Rather, they serve "as markers of friendly interaction ... and to emphasize intended statements of fact.... "[10]

The exclamation point has become popular in informal writing, where it efficiently functions as shorthand—*Thanks! Great! Perfect!*—that readily replaces a more protracted acknowledgment or thank you. Particularly in email correspondence, texting, tweeting, and Facebooking, an exclaimed word or phrase is seen as an acceptable and sufficient response by today's digital reader. And increasingly in informal contexts, the reader's expectations are such that a short message ending in anything other than an exclamation point may be viewed as chilly and distant.

PERIODS, QUESTION MARKS, AND EXCLAMATION POINTS: KEY DIFFERENCES BETWEEN AMERICAN AND BRITISH STYLE

Periods (what the British call *full stops*)

❖ *Oxford Style* omits the period (also referred to as a full point or a full stop) after abbreviations ending in the last letter of the abbreviated word; the British refer to these types of abbreviations as contractions.[11]

    apt ave Dr jr ltd Mr Mrs sr st (saint)

A period follows an abbreviation **not** ending in the last letter of the word abbreviated. (One notable exception: To distinguish *saint* from *street*, the former is abbreviated without a period—*st*; the latter is abbreviated with a period—*st.*)[12]

    ch. ed. etc. misc. Rev. (or Revd) no. vol.

According to *Oxford Style*: "A problem can arise with plural forms of abbreviations such as *vol.* (volume) or *ch.* (chapter): these would strictly be *vols* and *chs*, which are contractions and should **not** end with a point. However, this can lead to the inconsistent-looking juxtaposition of *vol.* and *vols* or *ch.* and *chs*, and so in some styles full points are retained for all such short forms. Similarly, *Bros*, the plural form of *Bro.* 'brother', is often written with a point."[13]

❖ The days of the week and most months of the year, however, are abbreviated with periods.[14]

    Sun. Mon. Tues. Wed. Thur. Fri. Sat.
    Jan. Feb. Mar. Apr. May June July Aug. Sept. Oct.
    Nov. Dec.

❖ Some British publications capitalize only the first letter of an acronym. *Oxford Style* notes,

"In some house styles any all-capital proper-name acronym that may be pronounced as a word is written with a single initial capital, giving *Basic*, *Unesco*, *Unicef*, etc; some styles dictate that an acronym is written thus if it exceeds a certain number of letters (often four)."[15]

❖ Periods, **not** colons, are placed between the representation of hours and minutes.[16]

    6.30 a.m. 7.30 p.m. 12 a.m. 12 p.m. [twelve-hour clock]
    18.10 23.15 12.00 24.00 [twenty-four-hour clock]

Question Marks and Exclamation Points
(what the British call exclamation *marks*)

❖ *Oxford Style* does **not** endorse using double punctuation (even in cases *Chicago* now allows): "When the quoted sentence ends with a question mark or exclamation mark, this should be placed within the closing quotation mark, with no other mark outside the quotation mark—only one mark of terminal punctuation is needed."[17]

- Has anyone read 'Punctuation Must Be Taught in Kindergarten!'
- Drop everything immediately and read 'Can Mastery of the Semicolon Change Your Life?'

Notes

1 For an extended discussion of how to abbreviate terms specific to various disciplines, see *Chicago*, 571–616.)
2 Patricia T. O'Conner, *Woe Is I: The Grammarphobe's Guide to Better English in Plain English* (New York: Riverhead Books, 1996), 153.
3 *Chicago*, 411.
4 *Chicago*, 411.
5 Jeff Guo, "Stop. Using. Periods. Period.," *The Washington Post*, June 13, 2016.
6 Danielle N. Gunraj, et al., "Texting Insincerely: The Role of the Period in Text Messaging," *Computers in Human Behavior* 55 (2016): 1069.
7 David Crystal, quoted in Dan Bilefsky, "Period. Full Stop. Point. Whatever It's Called, It's Going Out of Style," *The New York Times*, June 9, 2016.
8 F. Scott Fitzgerald, quoted in Sheilah Graham and Gerold Frank, *Beloved Infidel: The Education of a Woman* (New York: Henry Holt and Company, 1958), 198.
9 Leonard Elmore, *Elmore Leonard's 10 Rules of Writing*, illus. Joe Ciardiello (New York: William Morrow, 2007), 33.
10 Carol Waseleski, "Gender and the Use of Exclamation Points in Computer-Mediated Communication: An Analysis of Exclamations Posted to Two Electronic Discussion Lists," *Journal of Computer-Mediated Communication* 11, no. 4 (July 2006): 1020.
11 *Oxford Style*, 174, 176.
12 *Oxford Style*, 176, 179.
13 *Oxford Style*, 176.
14 *Oxford Style*, 179.
15 *Oxford Style*, 178.
16 *Oxford Style*, 194–95.
17 *Oxford Style*, 164.

2

COMMAS

Purpose and Application

By far, the comma is the most difficult form of punctuation to master because it serves several purposes; the rules governing its use can be difficult to apply, even when you know the rules; and some sentences require an added comma to avoid confusion, despite there being **no** formal rule for its addition. The comma plays a key role in aiding readability and minimizing confusion.

Separating Independent Clauses

2.1 Use a comma and a coordinating conjunction to join two independent clauses. Recall that an **independent clause** is a related word grouping that can stand alone as a *complete sentence* because it (a) includes a subject and predicate and (b) expresses a complete thought. A **dependent** (or **subordinate**) **clause** contains a subject and a predicate, but it does **not** express a complete thought. (*Incomplete sentences* are words and word groupings that, while ending in periods, question marks, or exclamation points, are missing a subject or a verb, or they do **not** express a complete thought.) The seven **coordinating conjunctions** are *and*, *but*, *for*, *or*, *nor*, *so*, and *yet*. One way to remember them is by the acronym FANBOYS.

- I like what Theodore Bernstein says about writing,[1] and I love what H. W. Fowler says about writing.[2]
- I like what Theodore Bernstein says about writing, but I love what H. W. Fowler says about writing.
- I like what Theodore Bernstein says about writing, for he seems to make a lot of sense.
- I plan on reading what Theodore Bernstein says about writing, or I may just re-read what H. W. Fowler says about writing.

- I do not like what Theodore Bernstein says about writing, nor do I like what H.W. Fowler says about writing.
- I love what H.W. Fowler says about writing, so I have recommended him to my friends.
- I love what H.W. Fowler says about writing, yet I don't agree with everything he says.
- Disappointed with my writing skills, my thesis advisor commanded: Attend every campus-sponsored writing workshop on academic writing held over the course of the academic year, and compile an annotated list of books you think might be helpful in improving your writing skills. [This is an example of an **imperative sentence**. It commands the subject (you), who is implied, to do something. The sentence includes two commands, both of which are treated as independent clauses despite neither having a stated subject.]

2.2 When you do **not** use a comma and coordinating conjunction, or other appropriate punctuation, to connect two independent clauses, a run-on sentence results. A **run-on sentence**, which is more difficult to read because it runs together ideas without benefit of any separating pause, can take one of two forms. A **fused sentence** includes **no** punctuation between independent clauses.

INCORRECT I like what Bernstein says about writing I love what Fowler says about writing.

Other times, the run-on sentence reflects what is called a **comma splice,** which is when you use a comma to splice or join two independent clauses.

INCORRECT I like what Bernstein says about writing, I love what Fowler says about writing.

Sometimes a run-on sentence can be challenging for a beginning writer to spot when the independent clauses seemingly flow together, as seen in the examples below. The first three run-ons are fused sentences; the fourth and fifth are comma splices.

INCORRECT I will be completely blunt *I am a horrible writer.*
INCORRECT I like writing *in fact I have always liked it.*
INCORRECT Some students never take responsibility for their writing problems *instead they just blame others.*
INCORRECT He didn't have enough time to complete the assignment, *it was just too long and too hard.*
INCORRECT She didn't study for the exam very long, *she had to work a double shift the night before, besides it was just the first of five exams in the course.* [three independent clauses; two comma splices]

In addition to using a comma and coordinating conjunction to join two independent clauses, they can be correctly punctuated in other ways to avoid a run-on sentence. Two independent clauses can be made into two sentences, they can be separated by a semicolon (if they are closely related), or they can be revised so that one of the independent clauses becomes a dependent clause (for further discussion of these options and their rhetorical potential, see Chapter 3: 3.1).

- I like what Bernstein says about writing. I love what Fowler says about writing.
- I like what Bernstein says about writing; I love what Fowler says about writing.
- Although I like what Bernstein says about writing, I love what Fowler says about writing.

2.3 Do **not** add a comma before a coordinating conjunction that joins a compound predicate. (A **compound predicate** refers to two or more predicates having the same subject, referenced once, which are connected by a coordinating conjunction. _She_ [subject] _read books and wrote poetry_ [compound predicate].

INCORRECT I like reading Bernstein's writing lessons, and applying them to my own writing.

CORRECT I like reading Bernstein's writing lessons and applying them to my own writing.

INCORRECT I love what Fowler says about writing, and agree with everything he says.

CORRECT I love what Fowler says about writing and agree with everything he says.

INCORRECT I plan on reading what Bernstein says about writing, or just re-reading what Fowler says about writing.

CORRECT I plan on reading what Bernstein says about writing or just re-reading what Fowler says about writing.

Occasionally, a comma added before a coordinating conjunction that joins a compound predicate can enhance readability and/or prevent confusion when the introductory independent clause becomes lengthier and more complex.

- I am going to read more of Bernstein and Fowler because they have helped me to become a more thoughtful and critical writer, and apply more of their advice to my writing.
- I plan on reading what Bernstein, Fowler, and others such as Pinker, Dryer, Fish, Williams, and Norris have to say about writing, and applying the advice to my own writing.

2.4 When you join two independent clauses that are relatively short, ideationally related, and structurally balanced, you *may* exclude the comma before the coordinating conjunction if the sentence is still easy to read without the comma.

INCORRECT I like Bernstein but I love Fowler because he covers so much ground in so much detail. [comma needed after *Bernstein*]
CORRECT I like Bernstein but I love Fowler.
CORRECT I like Bernstein, but I love Fowler.
INCORRECT I like Bernstein and I love Fowler because he covers so much ground in so much detail. [comma needed after *Bernstein*]
CORRECT I like Bernstein and I love Fowler.
CORRECT I like Bernstein, and I love Fowler.

2.5 A comma splice is acceptable if its independent clauses are relatively short, ideationally related, and structurally balanced. In these rare cases, commas, instead of semicolons, are favored by authors wanting an even closer connection between the independent clauses. The effect is a more dramatic presentation of ideas.

- "I came, I saw, I conquered."[3]
- "It was the best of times, it was the worst of times."[4]
- "But these thoughts broke apart in his head and were replaced by strange fragments: This is my soul and the world unwinding, this is my heart in the still winter air."[5]

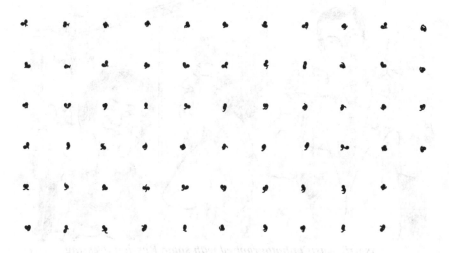

The Comma Sutra

PAUL
NOTH

2.6 Sometimes a comma splice makes sense—although **not** all would agree—if the second independent clause completes a "hanging thought" introduced by the first. *She wasn't dishonest, she was diplomatic.* Similarly, in the examples below—drawn mostly from journalism, where the practice appears more prevalently—the second independent clause juxtaposes with the first, and the semicolon that would normally have set off the two independent clauses is replaced with a comma, which more closely unites the two clauses.

- "Our struggle is not the struggle of a day, a week, a month, or a year, it is the struggle of a lifetime."[6]
- "Shadow is not my fur baby or my wife or my best friend, she's just a dog."[7]
- "For California, immigration is not an issue to be exploited to inflame hate and assuage the economic insecurities of those who feel displaced by the 21st-century economy, it's what keeps the state economy churning."[8]
- "The Lakers … aren't just old and awful at this point, they're injured too."[9]
- "Kirk Kerkorian, who died Monday at 98, wasn't just a fabulously rich corporate investor, he was an uncommon individual: intensely private, a billionaire with middle-class touches, a self-described 'gambler at heart.'"[10]

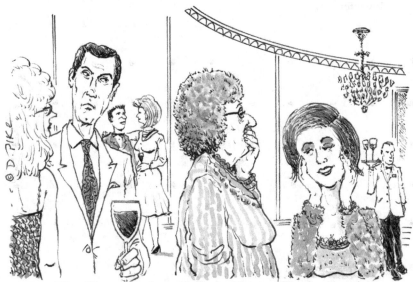

His wife wasn't photographed with some Russian dressing,
she was photographed with some Russian, dressing.

Pike, Doug; www.CartoonStock.com

Separating Items in a Series

2.7 Use a comma to separate three or more items in a series.

* Wilbur helped Beverly, Sylvia, and Buzz with their writing.
* Wilbur was asked by Beverly, Sylvia, and Buzz whether he wanted to be called a tutor, mentor, or coach.
* Wilbur taught Beverly, Sylvia, and Buzz how to write a thesis statement, structure a paper, and develop supporting arguments.
* Beverly, Sylvia, and Buzz came to understand that writing is hard work, writing requires an attention to detail, and rewriting is key to success.

The comma before the *and* (or before the *or*) is called a **serial** (or **series**) **comma** or the **Oxford comma**. Although some discussions of punctuation suggest the Oxford comma is optional, the vast majority of style manuals and composition texts now recommend using it to avoid the sort of potential reader confusion and writer embarrassment seen in these examples:

* "Among those interviewed were his two ex-wives, Kris Kristofferson and Robert Duvall."[11]
* "At the hotel Thursday afternoon, Houston drew the attention of reporters and security staff members with her erratic behavior, dripping sweat and disheveled clothes."[12]
* They liked fast cars, barbequed steaks and cats.
* He thanked his parents, Mary and God.
* She took a camping trip with her best friends, two Golden Retrievers and a third cousin.

Had a comma been added before the "and" in each sentence, it would have been clearer that Kris Kristofferson and Robert Duval are **not** ex-wives; Houston's erratic behavior was separate from, **not** exhibited by, her dripping sweat and disheveled clothes; cats are **not** being barbequed along with steaks; *he* is **not** Jesus; and her best friends are **not** two dogs and a third cousin.

Granted, the Oxford comma does **not** eliminate all ambiguity. Take the last example: *She took a camping trip with her best friends, two Golden Retrievers and a third cousin.* Even when a comma is placed after *Retrievers*, the meaning remains unclear. *She took a camping trip with her best friends, two Golden Retrievers, and a third cousin.* Is it now just her two Golden Retrievers that are her best friends? Revising the sentence eliminates any possibility of confusion: *She took a camping trip with her best friends, a third cousin, and two Golden Retrievers.*

Those arguing against the Oxford comma maintain it is unnecessary (i.e., a comma is the equivalent of saying *and*), interruptive, and wasteful of time and

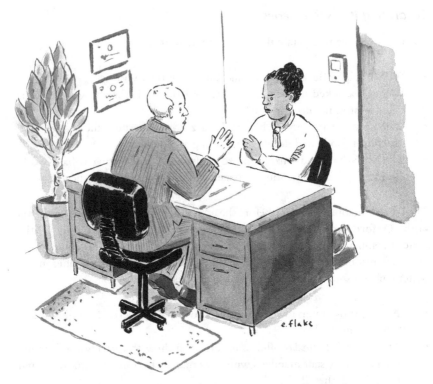

"I'm sorry, but refusing to use an Oxford comma isn't really grounds for divorce."

space; and in those cases where its absence could cause confusion, the sentence can easily be restructured. *They liked fast cars, barbequed steaks and cats* becomes *They liked fast cars, cats and barbequed steaks.* But the likelihood of such revision assumes that every writer will immediately recognize the culprit sentence before the final draft. In *Dryer's English: An Utterly Correct Guide to Clarity and Style,* Benjamin Dryer perhaps best summarizes the case for the Oxford comma: "No sentence has ever been harmed by a series comma, and many a sentence has been improved by one."[13] Certainly, as we are reminded by news stories from time to

AP STYLEBOOK, CHICAGO, APA, MLA, AND OXFORD STYLE

AP Stylebook shies away from the Oxford comma, excepting where the structure or complexity of the series is such that confusion would be averted by adding the Oxford comma.[15] *Chicago,* on the other hand, "strongly recommends"

always using the Oxford comma "since it prevents ambiguity."[16] *MLA*[17] and *APA*[18] recommend the same, as does *Oxford Style,* reminding the reader, "For a century it has been part of Oxford University Press style to retain or impose this last comma consistently, to the extent that the convention has also come to be called the **Oxford comma.**"[19]

time, **no** legal document has ever been harmed by a serial comma.[14] Suffice to say, the Oxford comma functions as a safeguard against potential embarrassment, ensuring the writer has one less thing to worry about.

2.8 Place a comma before *et cetera* (or *etc.*) when it completes a series. Do **not** add *and* before *et cetera* or *etc.* (Generally, *etc.* is used in less formal writing.) *Et cetera* means *and so forth.* To write *and et cetera* is redundant.

INCORRECT I shared rules, tips, advice, and et cetera for using punctuation effectively.
CORRECT I shared rules, tips, advice, et cetera for using punctuation effectively.
INCORRECT I shared rules, tips, advice, and etc. for using punctuation effectively.
CORRECT I shared rules, tips, advice, etc. for using punctuation effectively.

Likewise, *and* should **not** precede the abbreviation *et al.* (from the Latin *et alia,* meaning *and others*), which is used in reference citations.

2.9 Do **not** add a comma after the first item in a series having only two items.

INCORRECT Josie helped Sue, and Roger with their use of commas.
CORRECT Josie helped Sue and Roger with their use of commas.
INCORRECT Two of my favorite books are *Pause and Effect: An Introduction to the History of Punctuation in the West,* and *Making a Point: The Persnickety Story of English Punctuation.*
CORRECT Two of my favorite books are *Pause and Effect: An Introduction to the History of Punctuation in the West* and *Making a Point: The Persnickety Story of English Punctuation.*

2.10 Do **not** add a comma before the last item in a series if the item is preceded by an ampersand (&) instead of an *and* (unless you are following *APA*[20]). Although the ampersand is seldom used in narrative text, it commonly appears in book titles, film titles, and corporate names.

* *Shady Characters: The Secret Life of Punctuation, Symbols & Other Typographical Marks*
* *Legally Blond 2: Red, White & Blond*
* Blakely, Sokoloff, Taylor & Zafman, LLP

Separating Dependent Clauses

2.11 Place a comma after a dependent introductory clause when it comes before the main (independent) clause. Dependent (or subordinate) clauses begin with subordinating conjunctions, such as *after, although, as, because, before, even if, even though, if, since, so that, than, that, though, unless, until, when, whenever, where, whereas, wherever, whether, while*.

- After he took his eleventh creative writing course, her former husband decided he was ready to start his first short story.
- Although she never completed a creative writing class, she became an award-winning novelist.
- Because she was popular, she was frequently invited to speak at writing conferences.
- Before she even became successful, she pledged she would help other beginning writers in whatever ways she could.
- When she saw her former husband at writing conferences, she always asked how his writing was progressing.
- If he had been less of a jerk during their marriage, she would have made more of an effort to help him with his writing.
- Until the time came when she could forgive him, she would keep her interactions with him to a minimum.

2.12 Place a comma after an independent clause that is followed by a nonessential dependent clause. A **nonessential** (or **nonrestrictive**) element is one whose presence does **not** significantly affect the meaning of the sentence. When you set off a nonessential element with commas, you are saying that it can be omitted without major consequence to the meaning of the sentence. An **essential** (or **restrictive)** element, on the other hand, restricts or defines the meaning of what it modifies in the sense that the meaning would be unclear if the essential element were omitted. Because an essential element informs the meaning of the sentence, it cannot be set off by commas as if it were optional.

The distinction between essential and nonessential can be illustrated by taking the first two examples above and flipping their structure so that the independent clause now comes before the dependent clause. The dependent clause in the first example is essential; the dependent clause in the second example is nonessential.

- Her former husband decided he was ready to start his first short story after he took his eleventh creative writing course.
- She became an award-winning novelist, although she never completed a creative writing class

In the first example, it is essential to know when the husband started writing his first short story, a fact that forms the crux of the sentence. The essence of the second sentence, which tells us the former wife became an award-winning novelist, ends with *novelist*. If she ever completed a creative writing class may be interesting, but it is **not** essential to the meaning of the sentence.

Whether a clause is essential or nonessential is **not** always easy to determine. Complicating the decision is the fact that the same subordinating conjunction that begins an essential clause can also begin a nonessential clause.

- I will teach you how to use a comma if you will teach me how to use a semicolon.
- Could you please help me better understand what is meant by a nonessential clause, if you don't mind?
- I do well on exams when I study.
- I completed the exam, when my pen ran out of ink. [If, however, you meant to say that you somehow, miraculously, completed the exam only after your pen ran out of ink, the clause becomes essential, and **no** comma would follow *exam*.]
- It was hard to concentrate on studying for midterms while I awaited hearing whether my dog's surgery was successful.
- I studied for my test, while my dog took a nap on the sun porch.

Separating Adjectival Clauses

2.13 Use commas to set off a nonessential adjectival clause. An **adjectival clause** functions as an adjective. It modifies, in the sense of describing or clarifying, a noun or pronoun. An adjectival clause usually begins with a relative pronoun (*that, which, who, whom, whose*) and may be essential or nonessential. Compare these sentences:

- The professor who best exemplifies a commitment to students will win the Professor of the Year award.
- The newest member of the English Department, whom I have known since she was an undergraduate, won the Professor of the Year award.

In the first sentence, the modifying clause (*who best exemplifies a commitment to students*) is essential because it is central to the purpose of the sentence inasmuch as it defines who will win the award. In the second sentence, the modifying clause (*whom I have known since she was an undergraduate*) is nonessential because it does **not** affect the main idea expressed by the sentence, which would be true regardless of whether *I* had ever met the professor. *Who, whom,* and *whose* can be used to introduce essential and nonessential clauses.

When *that* and *which* are used, *that* introduces an essential clause and *which* usually introduces a nonessential clause. Some writers ignore the difference, perhaps bolstered by *Chicago*: "Although *which* can be substituted for *that* in a restrictive clause (a common practice in British English), many writers preserve the distinction. . . ."[21]

Below are two *that* examples where the adjectival clause is essential to the meaning of the sentence, followed by two *which* examples where the adjectival clause is nonessential.

- The speech that the mayor delivered at her inaugural ceremony was applauded by both political parties.
- The speech that the mayor gave on courageous leadership was viewed as one of her most eloquent presentations.
- The speech, which ran fifteen minutes, addressed the topic of climate control.
- The speech, which was broadcast live, was delivered in English and Spanish.

Separating Appositives

2.14 Use commas to set off a nonessential appositive. An **appositive** is a noun or noun phrase that renames, or defines, an adjacent noun or pronoun. An appositive can come at the beginning, middle, or end of a sentence, although it most commonly appears *after* a noun or pronoun. In the first four examples below, the appositives are nonessential to the meaning of the sentence, whereas in the last two examples they are essential.

- My English teacher, Mr. Wright, was seldom wrong. [*Mr. Wright* is nonessential, assuming you have only one English teacher.]
- Mr. Wright, the oldest faculty member in the school, was voted Most Popular Teacher.
- The most popular teacher in the school, Mr. Wright, was seldom wrong.
- The Most Popular Teacher award was given to Mr. Wright, my English teacher.
- The historian Doris Kearns Goodwin spoke at our campus.
- It was the teacher known as Mr. Composition who helped me most with my writing.

Whether an appositive is essential or nonessential depends on the facts informing the sentence. Both of these sentences, for example, could be correct:

- Glenn showered his wife Jane with expensive gifts.
- Glenn showered his wife, Jane, with expensive gifts.

The first sentence would be correct if Glenn has been married to more than one woman, because the sentence must reference a specific wife by name for the audience to know which wife received the expensive gifts. *Jane*, the specific wife, is essential and must appear in the sentence without being set off by commas. The second sentence, however, would be correct if Glenn has had only one wife. Eliminating *Jane* from the sentence would **not** affect its meaning because *wife* cannot refer to anyone other than Jane. (But when *wife* functions as an adjective, as in *Glenn showered wife Jane with expensive gifts*, **no** comma follows *wife*. This sentence, for example, would also be correct: *He is survived by his wife, Rebecca; children Alexander and Leah; brother Stephen; and sister Susan.*)

And should Glenn and Jane have one daughter, it would be correct to say that *Glenn and Jane's daughter, Victoria, loves talking about essential and nonessential modifiers.* But if Glenn and Jane have more than one daughter, *Victoria* becomes essential, and the sentence must be punctuated without commas. *Glenn and Jane's daughter Victoria loves talking about essential and nonessential modifiers.*

The difference between essential and nonessential explains why seemingly similar sentences are punctuated differently.

- Margaret Mitchell's bestselling novel, *Gone with the Wind*, should be required reading for every high school student.
- John Steinbeck's bestselling novel *The Grapes of Wrath* should be required reading for every high school student.

Because Mitchell wrote only one bestselling novel, *Gone with the Wind* is non-essential; it is the only novel to which *bestselling novel* can refer. Steinbeck, in contrast, wrote several bestsellers. If *The Grapes of Wrath* were omitted from the sentence, the reader would have **no** idea which bestselling Steinbeck novel the writer of the sentence had in mind. Both sentences are punctuated correctly. So are these:

- We read Steinbeck's novel *Of Mice and Men.*
- We read Steinbeck's first novel, *Cup of Gold.*
- Marla re-read her favorite Steinbeck novel, *East of Eden.* [The *favorite Steinbeck novel* referenced can only be one novel. *East of Eden* is thus nonessential even though the reader may **not** have known beforehand which novel was Marla's favorite.]
- Steinbeck's novel *East of Eden* is my favorite.

Separating Transitional Words and Phrases

2.15 Use a comma to separate an introductory transitional word or phrase from the rest of sentence. **Transitional words and phrases** help the reader by labeling and bridging the writer's sentences or the writer's thoughts within a sentence. Many transitional words are conjunctive adverbs. A **conjunctive adverb** shows the relationship between two or more sentences, two independent clauses within one sentence, or the ideas within one sentence. That relationship most often takes the form of comparison (*likewise, similarly*), contrast (*however, rather*), cause and effect (*consequently, therefore*), and sequence (*finally, subsequently*). Conjunctive adverbs can also indicate addition (*furthermore, moreover*), emphasis (*certainly, indeed*), and time (*meanwhile, now*). Examples of other popular conjunctive adverbs include *accordingly, also, besides, first, further, hence, instead, nevertheless, otherwise, still, surely, then, thus, too, undoubtedly*. When a conjunctive adverb comes at the beginning or end of a sentence, it is set off by a comma; when it comes in the middle of a sentence, it is preceded and followed by commas.

- However, any discussion of commas is complicated but still worth the effort.
- Any discussion of commas is complicated but still worth the effort, however.
- Any discussion of commas, however, is complicated but still worth the effort.

A comma is omitted after a conjunctive adverb if it helps complete the meaning of the sentence.

- They cheated on the punctuation test and *thus* received failing grades.
- They *subsequently* dropped out of school.
- Despite appearing nonchalant, they are *indeed* committed to improving their punctuation skills.

When a transitional phrase (such as *after all, as a consequence, as a result, as such, for example, for instance, in addition, in conclusion, in fact, in other words, in sum, in summary, of course, on the other hand, to be sure*) comes at the beginning or end of a sentence, it is set off by a comma; when it comes in the middle of a sentence, it is preceded and followed by commas.

- For example, let's discuss the importance of commas.
- Let's discuss, for example, the importance of commas.
- Let's discuss the importance of commas, for example.

Separating Introductory Adverbs

2.16 Place a comma after a sentence adverb, which refers to a type of adverb. An **adverb** can modify a verb, adjective, other adverb, and even an entire sentence. When modifying a verb, an adverb indicates when, where, how, how often, under what conditions, or why the action occurred. An adverb that modifies the sentence as a whole is called a **sentence adverb**. Usually coming at the beginning of the sentence, it reflects the writer's attitude towards the sentence's content. Often ending in *ly*, sentence adverbs include such adverbs as *actually, admittedly, apparently, basically, certainly, clearly, curiously, evidently, fortunately, frankly, ideally, interestingly, ironically, mercifully, naturally, obviously, oddly, personally, presumably, regrettably, surprisingly, thankfully, ultimately, unfortunately*.

- Curiously, the English teacher never taught any of her children about punctuation.
- Ironically, all her children now love punctuation.
- Fortunately, all her children still talk to their mom.
- Ideally, everyone should teach their children about punctuation.
- Naturally, I teach my children about punctuation.

When a sentence adverb appears in the middle of a sentence, it is set off by commas.

- The English teacher, curiously, never taught any of her children about punctuation.
- All her children, ironically, came to love punctuation.

Certain other adverbs (such as *historically, holistically, hypothetically, linguistically, paradoxically, parenthetically, politically, psychologically, sociologically, structurally, stylistically, technically*) are similar to sentence adverbs in the sense they provide modifying context for the whole sentence. They, too, should be followed by a comma when they begin a sentence.

2.17 When a sentence begins with an adverb that modifies the sentence's verb, a comma does **not** need to follow the adverb, although writers sometimes include the comma to pause the reader and emphasize the adverb.

- Often I study into the wee hours of the night.
- Sometimes I study into the wee hours of the night.
- Yesterday I studied into the wee hours of the night.
- Today I will study into the wee hours of the night.
- Tomorrow I will study into the wee hours of the night.

Even when an introductory adverb ends in *ly*, a comma afterwards is **not** necessary if the adverb does **not** modify the whole sentence. (It is common, however, to find writers choosing to set off every introductory adverb ending in *ly*, irrespective of whether it serves as a sentence adverb or as a conjunctive adverb.)

- Quickly I realized the importance of effective punctuation.
- Frequently I talk about the excitement of proper punctuation.
- Usually I spend most of my free time helping others with their punctuation.
- Recently I concluded I should teach social media punctuation practices.
- Eagerly I awaited teaching my next writing class.
- Occasionally I teach punctuation to prison inmates.

   But:

- Occasionally, deciding whether to place a comma after an introductory adverb can be a difficult decision. [Here, *occasionally* does **not** modify the sentence's verb in the sense that you occasionally decide (i.e., sometimes you choose to decide and sometimes you choose **not** to decide). Rather, it is the decision-making that is occasionally difficult. *Occasionally* thus functions as a sentence adverb.]

Separating Other Introductory Words

2.18 Use a comma to set off *yes/no* and similar-type responses, and words and phrases of direct address.

- Yes, I will mentor the debate team on proper punctuation.
- No, I will not mentor the debate team on appropriate phone etiquette.
- Sure, I will be happy to mentor the football team on proper punctuation.
- Okay, I can also mentor the basketball team.
- Well, it's not a problem.
- Elizabeth, call me and let know what you think of my new punctuation book.
- Please, Senator Warren, let me know what you think.
- My fellow Americans, can you do the same?

2.19 Place a comma after an adjective or participle that begins a sentence. A **participle** is a verb form ending in *ing* (present participle) or a verb form ending in *ed* or the past tense equivalent (past participle). Participles often function as adjectives.

- Aghast, she stared at her blind date as he trashed the Oxford comma.
- Unfazed, he kept talking.
- Moaning, she expressed her opposition without saying a word.
- Giggling, she thought about the worst dates she had ever endured.
- Exhausted, she fell asleep instantly once she got home.

2.20 Do **not** place a comma after a coordinating conjunction that begins a sentence, unless it is followed by material normally set off by commas.

- And I have chosen to work on mastering grammar as soon as I conquer punctuation.
- And, not surprisingly, I have chosen to work on mastering grammar as soon I conquer punctuation.
- But it is even more important to know how to write clearly and coherently.
- But, as my professor keeps reminding me, it is even more important to know how to write clearly and coherently.
- Yet some people believe that punctuation and grammar are not all that important.

- Yet, and I am not exaggerating, some people believe that punctuation and grammar are not all that important.

Separating Adverbial Phrases

2.21 Use a comma to separate an introductory adverbial phrase from the rest of the sentence. An **adverbial phrase** is a word grouping that functions as an adverb. Many adverbial phrases are **prepositional phrases**—phrases beginning with a **preposition** (such as *around, at, by, down, from, in, near, on, over, to, under, up, with*) and ending in a noun or noun equivalent—behaving as adverbs. Adverbial phrases can also take the form of **infinitive phrases**—phrases beginning with an **infinitive verb** (the word *to* followed by a verb in its simple form).

- After mastering punctuation, they set their sights on becoming proficient in grammar.
- Nearly every week, they met as a group to peer review their papers.
- Unless paid in advance, she would not give a speech on such short notice.
- Because of his attention to detail, he enjoyed discovering all the nuances of comma use.
- In high school and college, she excelled at writing.
- By reading and writing every day, they improved their critical thinking skills.
- With fanatical fixation, he dedicated himself to becoming less obsessive about punctuation.
- To master the nuances of comma use, she enlisted the help of The Comma Guru.
- To improve his punctuation skills, he joined the school's Punctuation Club.

2.22 When an adverbial phrase comes immediately after the subject but before the predicate, it is set off by commas.

- Bruce and Greg, after mastering punctuation, set their sights on becoming proficient in grammar.
- Bruce and Greg, nearly every week, met with their colleagues to discuss research projects.

2.23 When an adverbial phrase comes at the end of a sentence and is nonessential, it is set off by a comma.

- He worked on his memoir all the time, even on Super Bowl Sunday.
- He taught creative writing at a small liberal arts college, down the road from his childhood home.

The two sentences above contain both essential and nonessential adverbial clauses. In the first example, *all the time* is essential because it completes the thought, whereas *even on Super Bowl Sunday* is nonessential to completing that thought. In the second example, *at a small liberal arts college* is essential to the meaning of the sentence; *down the road from his childhood home* is nonessential.

2.24 When an adverbial clause comes at the end of a sentence and is essential, it is **not** set off by a comma.

- She did her best writing whenever pressured.
- He agreed to submit his recorded interviews if legally required.

2.25 You *may* omit a comma after a short introductory adverbial phrase, although it can be included (as seen throughout in the pages of this book).

- By next Friday I will know my grade.
  Or:
  By next Friday, I will know my grade
- In sum I did everything I could to succeed in the class.
  Or:
  In sum, I did everything I could to succeed in the class.
- If possible would you email me your comments on my paper?
  Or:
  If possible, would you email your comments on your paper?

If you choose to omit the comma, you will need to decide exactly how many words constitute a short phrase and then consistently apply the standard. And you will still need to add the comma in cases where its absence would cause confusion.

ORIGINAL After cooking the chef always prepared a special meal for himself.
REVISION After cooking, the chef always prepared a special meal for himself.
ORIGINAL Before meeting Bob Dylan was reading *Punctuation Revisited*.
REVISION Before meeting Bob, Dylan was reading *Punctuation Revisited*.

2.26 Do **not** place a comma after an adverbial phrase that begins an **inverted sentence**, which is a sentence whose verb comes before the subject.

- In front of a large and admiring crowd appeared the Prince of Punctuation.
- Behind the curtain waited the Princess of Punctuation.

Separating Participial Phrases

2.27 Use a comma to separate an introductory participial phrase from the rest of the sentence. A **participial phrase** is a word grouping, built around a participle, that modifies a noun or pronoun in much the same way an adjective would (by defining, qualifying, or quantifying).

- Recognizing his writing problems, he decided to enlist the help of a tutor.
- Frustrated by his writing problems, he decided to enlist the help of a tutor.

2.28 When a nonessential participial phrase comes in the middle of a sentence, it is set off by commas. **No** commas, however, should precede or follow an essential participial phrase.

- The student, discouraged by her study skills, sought the help of an academic counselor.
- Students discouraged by their study skills should seek the help of an academic counselor.

2.29 When a nonessential participial phrase comes at the end of a sentence, it is set off by commas. **No** commas, however, should precede or follow an essential participial phrase.

- She always worked diligently, appreciating the rewards of hard work.
- He spent countless hours tutoring anyone wanting to become a better writer.

Note: Unlike a participial phrase, a **gerund phrase** (a phrase that begins with a **gerund**, which is a noun formed by adding *ing* to a verb[22]) can function as the subject of the sentence. As such, **no** comma follows a gerund phrase when it begins a sentence and is followed by a verb.

- Recognizing his writing problems was something he initially tried to avoid.
- Finding the perfect writing coach would take time.

Separating Participial and Adverbial Phrases in a Compound Sentence

2.30 Use commas to set off an adverbial or participial phrase that appears within a compound sentence (a sentence having at least two independent clauses). A comma normally would precede the coordinating conjunction joining the two independent clauses.

- They improved their writing skills, and, after intensive tutoring, they enhanced their critical thinking skills.
- She liked him, but, knowing his many problems with punctuation, she hesitated to date him.

> ### CHICAGO
>
> Although it would **not** normally place a comma before the coordinating conjunctions (*and* in the first example; *but* in the second example) in the sentences above, *Chicago* acknowledges: "Strictly speaking, it would not be wrong.... Such usage, which would extend the logic of commas in pairs ... , may be preferred in certain cases for emphasis or clarity."[23]

Nonessential modifiers appearing *within* nonessential modifiers are normally also set off by commas.

> My best friend, who, until 2018, taught at the University of London, wrote a superb book about punctuation. [nonessential modifier: *who taught at the University of London*; nonessential modifier within a nonessential modifier: *until 2018*]

For the sake of readability, however, many writers choose to omit one or more commas in such constructions, believing that any additional commas, however correct, would disrupt the flow of the sentence (a view **not** necessarily endorsed here). They would alternatively punctuate the sentence above in one of two ways:

- My best friend who, until 2018, taught at the University of London, wrote a superb book about punctuation.
- My best friend, who until 2018 taught at the University of London, wrote a superb book about punctuation.

2.31 Do **not** place a comma before a coordinating conjunction that precedes an adverbial phrase or participial phrase appearing in a sentence having a compound predicate.

INCORRECT They improved their writing skills, and, after intensive tutoring, enhanced their critical thinking skills.

CORRECT They improved their writing skills and, after intensive tutoring, enhanced their critical thinking skills.

INCORRECT She liked him, but, knowing his many problems with punctuation, hesitated to date him.

CORRECT She liked him but, knowing his many problems with punctuation, hesitated to date him.

Separating Absolute Phrases

2.32 Use a comma to separate an **absolute phrase** (a noun or pronoun followed most often by a participial phrase) from the rest of the sentence; **no** comma, however, comes between the noun and the participle. An absolute phrase modifies the entire sentence.

INCORRECT His writing skills, having dramatically improved, Muhammad decided to become an English tutor.

CORRECT His writing skills having dramatically improved, Muhammad decided to become an English tutor.

INCORRECT Muhammad, his writing skills, having dramatically improved, decided to become an English tutor.

CORRECT Muhammad, his writing skills having dramatically improved, decided to become an English tutor.

INCORRECT Muhammad decided to become an English tutor, his writing skills, having dramatically improved.

CORRECT Muhammad decided to become an English tutor, his writing skills having dramatically improved.

Separating Coordinate Adjectives

2.33 Use commas to separate **coordinate adjectives**. Two or more adjectives are coordinate if you can change their order within the sentence, or join them by *and*, and the sentence still makes sense.

- She lives in an orange, two-story, older house.
- She lives in an older, orange, two-story house.
- She lives in two-story, older, orange house.
- She lives in an older and orange two-story house.

In each sentence above, the meaning conveyed remains unchanged; irrespective of the order in which they appear, each adjective—*orange, two-story,* and *older*—still modifies the noun *house*.

Adjectives are **cumulative** or **noncoordinate** when they do **not** *all* directly modify a noun or pronoun. Cumulative adjectives are **not** separated by commas because they represent one set of adjectives. For example:

The Teachers Museum includes several designer leather briefcases.

In this sentence, *leather* modifies *briefcases, designer* modifies *leather briefcases,* and *several* modifies *designer leather briefcases.* Unlike coordinate adjectives, the order of cumulative adjectives cannot be reversed and still make sense.

- The Teachers Museum includes leather designer several briefcases.
- The Teachers Museum includes leather several designer briefcases.
- The Teachers Museum includes designer leather several briefcases.
- The Teachers Museum includes designer several leather briefcases.

Or take this example: *The house featured a glossy white front door.* Here, *front* modifies *door*, *white* modifies *front door*, and *glossy* modifies *white front door*. For this sentence to make sense, the modifying adjectives must appear in the specific order they do because they are cumulative, not coordinate.

Separating Parenthetical Material

2.34 Use commas to set off parenthetical material that appears in the middle or at the end of a sentence. As opposed to parentheses and dashes, commas integrate the parenthetical material into the grammatical structure of the sentence (for a discussion of how dashes and parentheses/brackets can also set off parenthetical material, see Chapter 4: 4.14 and Chapter 8).

- They loved, really loved, using commas to set off material.
- Parenthetical comments, please remember, are not crucial to understanding the point of the sentence.
- They actually believe, seriously, that punctuation does not matter.
- Those who categorically dismiss the importance of punctuation are uninformed and, well, simply wrong.
  Or, if the previous sentence featured two independent clauses:
  Those who categorically dismiss the importance of punctuation are uninformed, and, well, they are simply wrong.
- They hold an odd view of punctuation, needless to say.
- My lifelong study of punctuation has been worth it, or maybe not.

RHETORICALLY SPEAKING

Choosing to subordinate material to parenthetical status is often a rhetorical decision that implicitly reflects your attitudes and values. Consider these three sentences:

- Ricky and Lucy attended the Punctuation Workshop.
- Ricky, as well as Lucy, attended the Punctuation Workshop.
- Ricky, in addition to Lucy, attended the Punctuation Workshop.

The first sentence treats Ricky and Lucy nearly equally as a compound subject; the second and third sentences emphasize Ricky's attendance, subordinating Lucy's to secondary, nonessential status. Which raises the obvious question: Why? Why should Lucy be as equally parenthetical as the nephew and assistant in the sentences below?

- Ricky, as well as the three-year-old nephew he was babysitting, attended the Punctuation Workshop.
- Ricky, as well as his assistant, Desi, attended the Punctuation workshop.

When an *as well as* clause is essential, it is not set off by a comma.

- Ricky and Lucy have mastered punctuation as well as grammar.
- Lucy knows punctuation as well as Ricky.

Separating Contrasting Material

2.35 Use commas to set off contrasting elements that appear in the beginning, middle, or end of a sentence.

- Unlike Donald, Consuela excelled at punctuating contrasting elements.
- Consuela, not Donald, excelled at punctuating contrasting elements.
- The one who excelled at punctuating contrasting elements was Consuela, not Donald.

Separating Direct Questions

2.36 Use a comma when introducing a direct question, the first word of which should be capitalized.

- Today's composition teachers must often address the question, How important is punctuation in the digital age?
- Often she would wonder, Why do I care so much about punctuation?
- So, What do you think of my punctuation book?

Note: A direct question can also be introduced by a colon, which some publications may prefer.

Separating Tag Questions

2.37 Use a comma before a **tag question**, which is a question that follows a statement, turning the statement into a question. Do **not** capitalize the first word of a tag question.

- You don't think I should charge the debate team members for mentoring them about punctuation, do you?
- Debate is a wonderful extracurricular activity, isn't it?
- You like debate, right?

Separating Indirect Quotations

2.38 Use commas to set off the source of an indirect quotation (in the form of a paraphrase) when attribution is given within a sentence.

• Teaching her students how to correctly punctuate indirect quotations, Professor Mills announced, would be her next mission.
• The success of that mission might take a while, she continually told herself.

(For a discussion of comma use with direct quotations, see Chapter 6: 6.2, 6.15).

Signifying Omitted Words

2.39 Use a comma to signify omitted words you expect to be filled in by the reader.

> In the end, many tennis players struggled with the intricacies and nuances of commas; others, with semicolons and colons; and some, with dashes and parentheses.

The commas after *others* and *some* take the place of *struggled with*, as in *others struggled with semicolons and dashes . . . some struggled with semicolons and dashes.*

Avoiding Confusion

2.40 Use a comma in constructions that might otherwise cause confusion or, worse, lower your credibility. Another option always, of course, is to restructure the sentence.

ORIGINAL The lion was finally able to run after the veterinarian performed hip replacement surgery.
REVISION The lion was finally able to run, after the veterinarian performed hip replacement surgery.
ORIGINAL The concerned doctor wanted to see the patient now and then occasionally.
REVISION The concerned doctor wanted to see the patient now, and then occasionally.
ORIGINAL For some service animals provide crucial access and freedom.
REVISION For some, service animals provide crucial access and freedom.
ORIGINAL Christian and Fatima have three girls and two boys from Christian's marriage.
REVISION Christian and Fatima have three girls, and two boys from Christian's first marriage.
ORIGINAL Those who can teach; those who cannot criticize.

REVISION Those who can, teach; those who cannot, criticize.
ORIGINAL I was amazed how well I fit in in the Protest Against Bad Punctuation.
REVISION I was amazed how well I fit in, in the Protest Against Bad Punctuation.

Separating Abbreviations

2.41 Place a comma after *i.e.* (from the Latin *id est*, meaning *that is*) and *e.g.* (from the Latin *exempli gratia*, meaning *for example*). In more formal writing, *i.e.* and *e.g.* are placed in parentheses along with the text that follows. In less formal writing, they run with the rest of the text.

- I also helped (i.e., somewhat improved) the punctuation skills of several football players, especially some on the offensive team (e.g., the quarterback and the center).
- I also helped, i.e., somewhat improved, the punctuation skills of several football players, especially some on the offensive team, e.g., the quarterback and the center.

2.42 Place a comma before and after an academic degree that follows a name.

   Jennifer Docktorit, PhD, met with Melanie Docktore, MD, to discuss their mutual interest in weird, similar-sounding names.

2.43 Do **not** place a comma before or after an abbreviated suffix (e.g., *Jr.* or *Sr.*) or a Roman numeral suffix (e.g., *II* or *III*) that follows a name. Nor does a comma precede or follow the abbreviations *Inc.* (incorporated) or *Ltd.* (limited company) when they follow a company name.

- Sean O'Sullivan Sr. and Sean O'Sullivan Jr. met with their favorite cousins, Ian O'Sullivan II and Ian O'Sullivan III, to gauge their interest in contributing to a proposed book on the history of suffixes.
- Punctuation Professionals Inc. is dedicated to serving the needs of Fortune 500 clients, while Pretty Punctuation Ltd. works primarily with entertainment industry talent.

Separating Elements in a Date

2.44 Use commas to set off the elements of a date. (A) Separate the month and day from the year, and the year from the rest of the sentence. (B) Separate the day of the week from the month and day, and the month and day from the rest of the text. (C) Separate the day of the week from the month and day, the month and day from the year, and the year from the rest of the text. (D) Separate the month and day from the rest of the text.

- June 20, 2019, was the day I met my punctuation soulmate. [A]
- Thursday, June 20, was the day I met my punctuation soulmate. [B]
- Thursday, June 20, 2019, was the day I met my punctuation soulmate. [C]
- We met on June 20, at the International Conference on Commas. [D]

Commas are **not** needed when the day comes before the month and year, a day does **not** precede the month and year, or a holiday comes in place of the day and month.

- We met on 20 June 2019 at the International Conference on Commas.
- We met in June 2019 and again in June 2020 at the International Conference on Commas.
- We met on Labor Day 2019 to discuss next year's International Conference on Commas.

When a date functions as an adjective, a comma does **not** need to follow the date.

- We met at the 2019 opening reception of the International Conference on Commas.
- We met at the June 2019 opening reception of the International Conference on Commas.
- We met at the June 20, 2019 opening reception of the International Conference on Commas.

CHICAGO

Chicago cautions that using a full date (one that includes the day, month, and year) as a descriptive adjective can sometimes be confusing: "If a full month-day-year date is used, then a comma is sometimes considered necessary both before and after the year {the May 27, 2016, ceremonies}. But this construction is awkward because the adjective (which is forward looking) contains two commas (which are backward looking); the construction is therefore best avoided {commencement ceremonies on May 27, 2016}."[24] The rewrite here makes it clear that the *number* of ceremonies was **not** 2016.

Separating Elements in an Address

2.45 Use commas to set off the elements of an address: separate the street from the city, and the city from the state. When you reference the city and state at the beginning or middle of a sentence, place a comma after the state to ensure that the city and state are set off from the rest of the text and correctly read as one entity. Do the same when referencing places whose names include a comma.

- Cal Poly Pomona is located at 3801 West Temple Avenue, Pomona, CA 91768.
- Pomona, California, is located about 30 miles east of Los Angeles, California.
- California State Polytechnic University, Pomona, is the official name for Cal Poly Pomona.

Do **not** place a comma between the state and the zip code. But do place a comma after the zip code if more information follows.

Send your comments and suggestions about *Punctuation Revisited* to Richard Kallan, Department of Communication, 3801 West Temple Avenue, Pomona, CA 91768, in an envelope, however large it may need to be.

Separating Numbers

2.46 Place a comma after each third digit, counting right to left, in numbers comprising four digits or more.

1,500 or 1500★   25,000   1,250,000   5,100,250,000

★Although style manuals recommend using a comma in four-digit numbers, it is **not** uncommon to find writers omitting the comma, sensing its absence does **not** affect readability. "In scientific writing," *Chicago* confirms, "commas are often omitted from four-digit numbers."[25]

2.47 Do **not** place commas in serial numbers, model numbers, various account numbers, street numbers, page numbers, social security numbers, telephone numbers, temperatures, and zip codes. Nor should commas be placed in the numbers following a decimal point (7.1425; never 7.1,425).

RHETORICALLY SPEAKING

No form of punctuation inspires more debate—and variation in usage—than the comma. That said, comma placement is by no means primarily subjective; in most instances, the correctness of using, or not using, a comma is generally agreed upon. Nevertheless, it is not always clear what is correct, let alone appropriate, punctuation for a specific situation.

The uniqueness of a sentence may invite adding a comma to enhance readability even though no rule calls for it, as shown in the examples above. At other times, adding an unrequired comma enriches the sentence's meaning, as seen in this description by David Brooks of how some people react to tragedy: "They seem to get smaller and more afraid, and never recover."[26] By pausing the reader after *afraid*, Brooks poignantly emphasizes that some *never recover*. On occasion, an added comma can also provide an enriching pause. "It was thoughtful and kind of you to offer this additional example, and very much appreciated."

Then, too, writers will sometimes omit a normally required comma whose absence, they believe, improves readability (see 2.30). Explains Pinker: "The rationale is that too many commas too close together can give a sentence a herky-jerky feel. Also, since a sentence may have many levels of branching while English provides only the puny comma to separate them all on the page, a writer may choose to keep the comma in reserve to demarcate the major branches in the tree, rather than dicing the sentence into many small pieces that the reader must then reassemble."[27]

On the other hand, commas, along with dashes, can create a rhythm that mimics a more conversational style, as Tom Wolfe demonstrates in his description of military pilots: "The world was used to enormous egos in artists, actors, entertainers of all sorts, in politicians, sport figures, and even journalists, because they had such familiar and convenient ways to show them off. But that slim young man over there in uniform, with the enormous watch on his wrist and the withdrawn look on his face, that young officer who is so shy that he can't even open his mouth unless the subject is flying—that young pilot—well, my friends, his ego is even *bigger!*—so big, it's *breathtaking!*"[28]

Notes

1 Theodore M. Bernstein's major works include *Watch Your Language: A Lively, Informal Guide to Better Writing, Emanating from the News Room of The New York Times* (Manhasset, New York: Channel Press, 1958); *The Careful Writer: A Modern Guide to English Usage* (New York: Atheneum, 1965); and *Miss Thistlebottom's Hobgoblins: The Careful Writer's Guide to the Taboos, Bugbears and Outmoded Rules of English Usage* (New York: Farrar, Straus and Giroux, 1971).
2 H.W. Fowler's classic work, *A Dictionary of Modern English Usage* (Oxford: Oxford University Press) was first published in 1926. The second edition, revised and edited by Sir Ernest Gowers, appeared in 1965. The third edition, retitled *The New Fowler's Modern English Usage* and edited by R.W. Burchfield, was published in 1996. In 2015, Oxford released the fourth and latest edition, *Fowler's Dictionary of Modern Usage*, edited by Jeremy Butterfield.

3 Julius Caesar, quoted in Suetonius, *History of Twelve Caesars,* trans. Philemon Holland, vol. 1 (London: David Nutt in the Strand, 1899), 42. Reprint of C. Suetonius Tranquillus, *The Historie of Twelve Caesars,* trans. Philemon Holland, 1606.

4 Charles Dickens, *The Tale of Two Cities,* illus. H. K. Browne (London: Chapman and Hall, 1859), 1. The example cited is an abridgement of the novel's opening series of run-on independent clauses.

5 Emily St. John Mandel, *Station Eleven* (New York: Knopf, 2014), 194.

6 John Lewis (@repjohnlewis), Twitter, June 27, 2018, 8:15 a.m., https:twitter.com/johnlewis/status/1011991303599607808?lang=en.

7 Maeve Higgins, "Get Yourself a Giant Dog," *The New York Times,* July 15, 2018.

8 Steve Kettman, "The Californization of American Politics," *The New York Times,* June 3, 2018.

9 Mike Bresnahan, "Lakers Leave Fans Unfulfilled," *Los Angeles Times,* January 7, 2013.

10 James F. Peltz, "Notable Chapters in the Life of a 'Born Gambler,'" *Los Angeles Times,* June 17, 2015.

11 Randy Lewis, "Haggard—Candid as Ever," *Los Angeles Times,* July 21, 2010. (Quotation appears in a photo caption accompanying the article.)

12 Geoff Boucher, "A Pop Superstar Turned Supernova," *Los Angeles Times,* February 12, 2012.

13 Benjamin Dryer, *Dryer's English: An Utterly Correct Guide to Clarity and Style* (New York: Random House, 2019), 24. According to Dryer, "Only godless savages eschew the series comma," p. 24.

14 See, for example, Daniel Victor, "A Judge, a Lawsuit and One Very Important Comma," *The New York Times,* March 17, 2017.

15 *AP Stylebook,* 322.

16 *Chicago,* 371.

17 *MLA,* 7th ed., 67.

18 *APA,* 88.

19 *Oxford Style,* 77.

20 *APA,* 175, 184.

21 *Chicago,* 376–77.

22 In other words, a gerund is a present participle that functions as a noun.

23 *Chicago,* 376; see also 375, 379–80.

24 *Chicago,* 252.

25 *Chicago,* 563.

26 David Brooks, "The Moral Peril of Meritocracy," *The New York Times,* April 7, 2019.

27 Pinker, *The Sense of Style,* 287.

28 Tom Wolfe, *The Right Stuff* (New York: Farrar, Straus and Giroux, 1979), 39.

3

SEMICOLONS

Purpose and Application

Providing more pause than a comma does but less than a period affords, a semicolon connects closely related independent clauses and, conversely, separates items in a series having internal punctuation. The most common semicolon fault is using it incorrectly in place of a comma.

Connecting Related Independent Clauses

3.1 A semicolon can connect two or more closely related independent clauses (see Chapter 1, Quick Reference Glossary). The independent clause that follows the semicolon is **not** capitalized.

- My older brother loves semicolons. [a sentence with one independent clause]
- My older brother loves semicolons; my younger brother hates them. [a sentence with two independent clauses]
- My older brother loves semicolons; my younger brother hates them; my twin sister has a love-hate relationship with them, semicolons that is. [a sentence with three independent clauses]

A semicolon bonds complementary independent clauses that represent a larger thought having two or more parts. Take the second bulleted example above: *My older brother loves semicolons; my younger brother hates them.* Pairing the two independent clauses with a semicolon and running them side-by-side using parallel

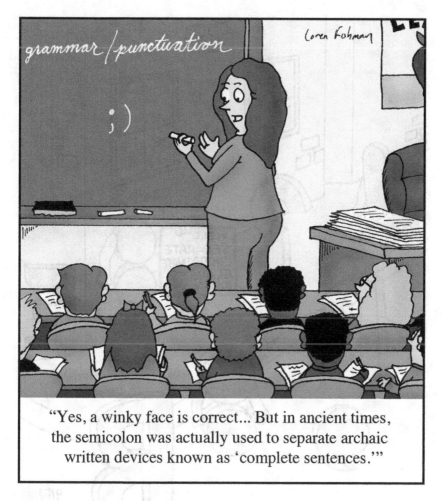

"Yes, a winky face is correct... But in ancient times, the semicolon was actually used to separate archaic written devices known as 'complete sentences.'"

Fishman, Loren; www.CartoonStock.com

language emphasizes the differences between the two brothers, which is the main point of the sentence.

Another option would be to link the two clauses with a comma and a coordinating conjunction—*and, but, for, or, nor, so, yet* (see Chapter 2: 2.1). But the impact of the sentence would **not** be the same: the intervening coordinating conjunction, such as *but* or *yet*, would slightly offset the parallelism of the comparison, diminishing its strength and elegance.

- My older brother loves semicolons, but my younger brother hates them.
- My older brother loves semicolons, yet my younger brother hates them.

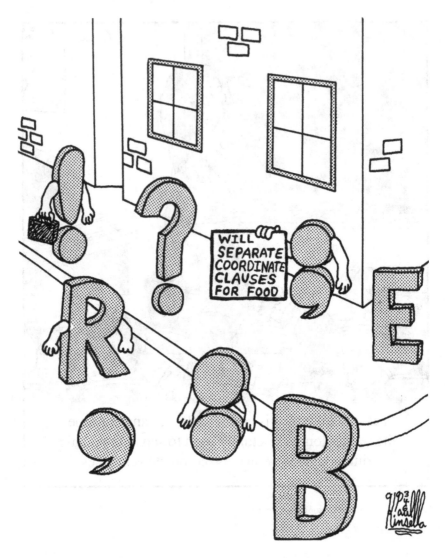

Kinsella, Paul; www.CartoonStock.com

The sample sentence can also be turned into two sentences, or it can be revised so that one of its independent clauses becomes dependent, which then structurally emphasizes the idea expressed in the lone independent clause.

- My older brother loves semicolons. My younger brother hates them.
- Although my older brother loves semicolons, my younger brother hates them.
  Or:
  My younger brother hates semicolons, although my older brother loves them.

But again, these options, although punctuationally correct, detract from the comparison and slightly change the meaning because they structurally separate the clauses to a greater degree than would a semicolon, which allows for closer pairing and a more direct comparison.

In *How to Write a Sentence: And How to Read One*, Stanley Fish provides us with another example of the effective use of the semicolon when he discloses: "Some appreciate fine art; others appreciate fine wines. I appreciate fine sentences."[1] Here, the first sentence joins two complementary ideas describing what people appreciate, followed by a contrasting sentence about what Fish appreciates. Fish's praise of fine sentences could have taken a different structure.

- Some appreciate fine art. Others appreciate fine wines. I appreciate fine sentences.
- Some appreciate fine art, and others appreciate fine wines. I appreciate fine sentences.

Neither of these two alternative versions (both correctly punctuated), however, quite captures the tone and tenor of Fish's original passage.

Short of revising your entire sentence, sometimes *only* a semicolon can effectively join two independent clauses. In the examples below, a comma and coordinating conjunction cannot easily substitute for the semicolon.

- "Well, in most people's experience, sentences don't exactly diagram themselves; they have to be coaxed, if not rassled."[2]
- "A writer who can handle a long sentence gracefully lets us take a breath at reasonable intervals and at appropriate places; one part of the sentence will echo another with coordinated and parallel elements."[3]
- "But I must say I have great respect for the semicolon; it's a very useful little chap."[4]
- "For the colon and dash, the second sentence is usually an example or elaboration; for the semicolon, the second sentence is usually a similar or opposite idea (as in this sentence)."[5]
- "A colon is sometimes preferable to a semicolon if the thrust of the sentence is forward: you are amplifying something, providing a definition or a list or an illustration. The semicolon sets up a different relationship; whatever follows relates in a more subtle way to what came before."[6]

RHETORICALLY SPEAKING

The semicolon, like all forms of punctuation, is simply a tool. It does not by itself magically produce closely related clauses that share a larger, collective meaning; the semicolon merely joins those clauses in a way that emphasizes their connection. Nor does the semicolon by itself create the balance and grace brought about when well-written, closely related clauses share the same stage.

Using a semicolon to separate two independent clauses is not categorially superior to separating the clauses with a comma and coordinating conjunction, opting for two separate sentences, or revising the sentence to include a dependent clause. The meaning you wish to convey determines the appropriate sentence structure and corresponding punctuation. In some cases, a sentence having two independent clauses joined by a semicolon is the best choice; in other instances, it is not.

3.2 A semicolon can connect two independent clauses when the second begins with a conjunctive adverb (see Chapter 2: 2.15). Writers often incorrectly try to connect such clauses by placing a comma before the conjunctive adverb, as if it were a coordinating conjunction. This results in a comma splice (see Chapter 2: 2.2), as illustrated by the following sentences:

INCORRECT I am not a good writer, however I know how to use semicolons.
INCORRECT I am a good writer, therefore I know how to use semicolons.
INCORRECT I am a good writer, consequently I know how to use semicolons.
INCORRECT I am a good writer, hence I know how to use semicolons.
INCORRECT I am a good writer, moreover I know how to use semicolons.

To revise these sentences (and various others whose second independent clause similarly begins with a conjunctive adverb, such as *accordingly, also, besides, certainly, consequently, finally, first, further, furthermore, hence, however, indeed, instead, likewise, meanwhile, moreover, nevertheless, now, otherwise, rather, similarly, still, subsequently, surely, then, thus, therefore, too, undoubtedly, yet*), delete the comma preceding the conjunctive adverb, replace it with a semicolon, and then add a comma after the conjunctive adverb.

CORRECT I am not a good writer; however, I know how to use semicolons.
        Or:
        I am not a good writer; I know how to use semicolons, however.
CORRECT I am a good writer; therefore, I know how to use semicolons.
CORRECT I am a good writer; consequently, I know how to use semicolons.
CORRECT I am a good writer; hence, I know how to use semicolons.
CORRECT I am a good writer; moreover, I know how to use semicolons.

3.3 Like conjunctive adverbs, transitional phrases (see Chapter 2: 2.15) cannot join two independent clauses unless preceded by a semicolon. Using only a comma creates a comma splice.

INCORRECT I know how to use a semicolon, in fact it's my favorite punctuation mark.

CORRECT I know how to use a semicolon; in fact, it's my favorite punctuation mark.

INCORRECT I know how to use a semicolon, for example I just used one.

CORRECT I know how to use a semicolon; for example, I just used one.

INCORRECT I know how to use a semicolon, in addition I know how to use a colon.

CORRECT I know how to use a semicolon; in addition, I know how to use a colon.

3.4 Use a semicolon before a coordinating conjunction (a) if the independent clause that precedes or follows the coordinating conjunction includes internal punctuation, (b) the clauses mandate greater separation because of their length and structure, or (c) you wish to emphasize the antithesis or contrast between the two clauses.

- In college, where she honed her writing skills, she learned the rules of punctuation, grammar, and usage, so she could express her ideas clearly, concisely, and compellingly; and she became a more critical reader, which would prove just as beneficial in her quest to become a famous author.
- Despite repeated requests, they refused to show any of their previously graded papers to the staff at the Tutorial Center, supposedly because they did poorly on all their writing assignments and needed everyone's full attention to pass their classes; or, on the other hand, maybe they were just exaggerating about their writing problems so they could get additional tutoring they might not otherwise receive given the pressing workload of the Tutorial Center.
- They were taught every form of punctuation again and again from the time they entered high school until they graduated college; but they mastered none until they went to prison.

A comma, instead of a semicolon, before the coordinating conjunction would have been technically correct in any of the above examples. The semicolon, however, renders each sentence easier to read by providing greater pause between the independent clauses.

CHICAGO

When connecting two independent clauses one of which includes internal punctuation, *Chicago* recommends using a semicolon before the coordinating conjunction only when the *second* clause has internal punctuation.[7]

RHETORICALLY SPEAKING

To be sure, a strategically placed semicolon can significantly enhance meaning. Mary Norris describes the semicolon as having "a vestigial inter-rogative quality to it, a cue to the reader that the writer is not finished yet; she is holding her breath."[8] Recalling her days as copyeditor, Norris considers what she would have done had she been reading dialogue and come across this sentence: "She looked at me; I was lost for words."[9] Norris says she would have been "tempted to poke in a period and make it into two sentences. In general, people—even people in love—do not speak in flights that demand semicolons. But in this instance, I have to admit that without the semicolon something would be lost. With a period, the four words sink at the end: SHE LOOKED at me. The semicolon keeps the words above water: because of that semicolon, something about her look is going to be significant."[10]

Separating Items in a Series

3.5 Use a semicolon to separate a series of main items when one or more of those items contains internal punctuation.

- Mark likes dogs, especially those belonging to the sporting, nonsporting, and working groups and if the dogs like rabbits; cats, if they are well behaved, which they usually are, except for the last one he adopted; birds; horses, but only if they are Arabians, Appaloosas, or Clydesdales, and they get along with dogs, cats, and birds; rabbits; and turtles.
- Candice likes dogs because they are affectionate, loyal, and protective, and she feels safe in their presence; cats because they are independent and save her a lot of money by ridding her seven homes of mice and other rodents; and horses because she lives in the country and can always count on them as an alternative form of transportation.
- My 8th grade girlfriend always wanted to talk about punctuation, especially commas, colons, and dashes; grammar, in particular subject–verb agreement, pronoun–antecedent agreement, and nominative versus objective case; usage; and mechanics, although she personally never liked to capitalize, italicize, or hyphenate anything.
- My 8th grade girlfriend dumped me when she realized four things: my knowl-edge of punctuation was restricted to periods, question marks, and exclama-tion points; my writing contained grammatical mistakes, such as using plural

pronouns with singular referents; I thought *usage* referred to drugs; and I only talked about *mechanics* in the context of shooting free throws.

In these examples, the semicolon provides a longer pause than would a comma, thereby aiding the reader in distinguishing between main items and the elaborative information specific to each item. The semicolon also functions to visually separate the main items, letting the reader instantly know where one ends and another begins.

Note: When a listed item contains internal punctuation, a semicolon follows *each* item in the list even if the item does **not** include internal punctuation; the punctuation that separates one item from another cannot be a combination of commas and semicolons.

Note: The last item in a series separated by semicolons must include a **serial semicolon** before the *and* that precedes the last item, as seen in the bulleted examples above. You would **not** want to omit a semicolon, for instance, after *rodents* in this previous example:

> Candice likes dogs because they are affectionate, loyal, and protective, and she feels safe in their presence; cats because they are independent and save her a lot of money by ridding her seven homes of mice and other rodents and horses because she lives in the country and can always count on them as an alternative form of transportation.

RHETORICALLY SPEAKING

Another option for separating items in a series, aside from commas (and, if necessary, semicolons), is to use bullets, which have the advantage of visually highlighting the listed items. Bullets are commonplace in informal writing, but less acceptable in formal venues, such as academic writing.

A bulleted list whose items do not contain internal punctuation can be formatted in one of two ways: with punctuation or without.

Our spy pens come in four colors:	*Or:*	*Our spy pens come in four colors:*
• black		• black,
• grey		• grey,
• grey and black		• grey and black, and
• black and white		• black and white.

A bulleted list whose items *do* contain internal punctuation can be punctuated in two ways:

Our spy pens come in four colors:	Or:	*Our spy pens come in four colors:*
• black, with red, green, and yellow highlights		• black, with red, green, and yellow highlights;
• grey, with red, green, and yellow highlights		• grey, with red, green, and yellow highlights;
• grey and black, with red, green, and yellow highlights		• grey and black, with red, green, and yellow highlights; and
• black and white, with red, green, and yellow highlights		• black and white, with red, green, and yellow highlights.

When the bulleted items comprise complete sentences, they must be followed by ending punctuation.

Good professors usually possess three qualities:

- They are knowledgeable.
- They are conscientious.
- They are accessible.

Adapted from Richard Kallan, *Renovating Your Writing: Shaping Ideas and Arguments into Clear, Concise, and Compelling Messages,* 2nd ed., Routledge, 2018. Permission courtesy of Routledge.

Eliminating Incorrect Semicolon Use

3.6 Do **not** place a semicolon between an independent clause, regardless of its length, and a dependent clause. Recall that a dependent or subordinate clause is a word grouping that while containing a subject and a predicate cannot stand alone as a (complete) sentence because it does **not** express a complete thought. Dependent clauses begin with subordinating conjunctions, such as *after, although, as, because, before, even if, even though, if, since, so that, than, that, though, unless, until, when, whenever, where, whereas, wherever, whether, while.* In the examples below, the independent clause (*I still have a long way to go to become an excellent writer*) is either preceded or followed by a dependent clause (*although I have worked steadfastly on improving my punctuation and becoming more proficient in grammar, mechanics, and usage*). A comma, **not** a semicolon, should separate the two clauses.

INCORRECT Although I have worked steadfastly on improving my punctuation and becoming more proficient in grammar, usage, and mechanics so that I might receive better grades on my term papers and essay exams; I still have a long way to go to become an excellent writer.

CORRECT Although I have worked steadfastly on improving my punctuation and becoming more proficient in grammar, usage, and mechanics so that I might receive better grades on my term papers and essay exams, I still have a long way to go to become an excellent writer.

INCORRECT I still have a long way to go to become an excellent writer; although I have worked steadfastly on improving my punctuation and becoming more proficient in grammar, usage, and mechanics so that I might receive better grades on my term papers and essay exams.

CORRECT I still have a long way to go to become an excellent writer, although I have worked steadfastly on improving my punctuation and becoming more proficient in grammar, usage, and mechanics so that I might receive better grades on my term papers and essay exams. [The dependent clause in this example (*although I have worked ...*) is preceded by a comma because it is nonessential (nonrestrictive).]

3.7 Do **not** place a semicolon after a conjunctive adverb used to introduce an independent clause.

INCORRECT I never thought I would come to appreciate semicolons. However; I could not have been any more wrong. Consequently; I find myself using them all the time, in almost every sentence I write. Therefore; I am now trying to limit myself to no more than five per page.

CORRECT I never thought I would come to appreciate semicolons. However, I could not have been any more wrong. Consequently, I find myself using them all the time, in almost every sentence I write. Therefore, I am now trying to limit myself to no more than five per page.

3.8 Do **not** place a semicolon after a salutation.

INCORRECT Dear Ms. Winfrey;
INCORRECT Dear Oprah;

Depending of the formality of the salutation, either a colon or a comma suffices.

CORRECT Dear Ms. Winfrey:
CORRECT Dear Oprah,

3.9 Do **not** place semicolons after each name in a multi-name salutation.

INCORRECT Dear Mr. Singh; Ms. Patel; and Friends of Mr. Singh and Ms. Patel:
CORRECT Dear Mr. Singh, Ms. Patel, and Friends of Mr. Singh and Ms. Patel:

3.10 Do **not** use a semicolon to introduce a list.

INCORRECT Their writing showed improvement in four areas; grammar, punctuation, usage, and mechanics.

CORRECT Their writing showed improvement in four areas: grammar, punctuation, usage, and mechanics.

3.11 Do **not** use semicolons to separate listed items introduced by a colon if none of the items include internal punctuation.

INCORRECT My favorite forms of punctuation are the following: colons; dashes; and semicolons.

CORRECT My favorite forms of punctuation are the following: colons, dashes, and semicolons.

INCORRECT Every night before I go to bed, I reread portions from three of my favorite books: *The Chicago Manual of Style*; *MLA Handbook for Writers of Research Papers*; and *Publication Manual of the American Psychological Association*.

CORRECT Every night before I go to bed, I reread portions from three of my favorite books: *The Chicago Manual of Style*, *MLA Handbook for Writers of Research Papers*, and *Publication Manual of the American Psychological Association*.

Use semicolons, **not** commas, however, when one or more items following a colon include internal punctuation (see 3.5).

RHETORICALLY SPEAKING

No form of punctuation has been more derided than the semicolon. Novelists and journalists have led the criticism. Kurt Vonnegut unabashedly declares: "Here is a lesson in creative writing. First rule: Do not use semicolons.... All they do is show you've been to college."[11] Bill Walsh, a former chief copy editor at the *Washington Post*, similarly berates the function of the semicolon in *Lapsing into a Coma: A Curmudgeon's Guide to Many Things That Can Go Wrong in Print—and How to Avoid Them*: "The semicolon is an ugly bastard, and thus I tend to avoid it. Its utility in patching together two closely related sentences is to be admired, but patches like that should be a make-do solution, to be used when nothing better comes to mind."[12]

Although Vonnegut and Walsh obviously overstate their case, creative writers and journalists, owing to the nature and of their storytelling, *do* build fewer sentence structures inviting of the semicolon. In contrast, other forms of expression—notably academic writing—frequently feature nuanced description and argument that mandate the kind of coordinated and sophisticated sentence structures enhanced by the semicolon, which explains why the mark is so appealing to academics, essayists, and critics.[13]

RHETORICALLY SPEAKING

The semicolon has been appropriated as a symbol of empowerment. Project Semicolon, a movement founded by Amy Bleuel in 2013, has as its mission "to help reduce the incidents of suicide in the world through connected community and greater access to information and resources."[14] According to Bleuel: "The project was started by asking others to draw a semicolon on their wrist to show support. The semicolon was chosen because in literature a semicolon is used when an author chooses to not end a sentence. You are the author and the sentence is your life. You are choosing to continue."[15] Today, many supporters of Project Semicolon exhibit the semicolon as a tattoo.

Notes

1 Stanley Fish, *How to Write a Sentence and How to Read One* (New York: HarperCollins, 2011), 3.
2 Kitty Burns Florey, *Sister Bernadette's Barking Dog: The Quirky History and Lost Art of Diagramming Sentences* (Hoboken, NJ: Melville House, 2006), 73.
3 Joseph M. Williams, *Style: Toward Clarity and Grace* (Chicago: University of Chicago Press, 1990), 143.
4 Abraham Lincoln, quoted in Noah Brooks, "Personal Reminiscences of Lincoln," *Scribner's Monthly, An Illustrated Magazine For the People*, February 1878, 566.
5 Edward P. Bailey, Jr., *The Plain English Approach to Business Writing*, rev. ed. (New York: Oxford University Press, 1997), 65.
6 Mary Norris, *Between You & Me: Confessions of a Comma Queen* (New York: W.W. Norton & Company, 2015), 145.
7 *Chicago*, 390.
8 Mary Norris, "Semicolons; So Tricky," *The New Yorker*, July 19, 2012, https://www.newyorker.com/books/page-turner/semicolons-so-tricky.
9 The sentence appeared in Thomas Bohm, *Punctuation. . ?*, 2nd ed. (Leicester, UK: User Design, 2012), 34.
10 Norris, "Semicolons; So Tricky."
11 Kurt Vonnegut, *A Man without a Country*, ed. Daniel Simon (New York: Seven Stories Press, 2005), 23.

12 Bill Walsh, *Lapsing into a Comma: A Curmudgeon's Guide to the Many Things That Can Go Wrong in Print—and How to Avoid Them* (New York: Contemporary Books, 2000), 91.

13 For a thoughtful defense of the semicolon, see Cecelia Watson, *Semicolon: The Past, Present, and Future of a Misunderstood Mark* (New York: Ecco, 2019).

14 Project Semicolon (website), accessed March 9, 2019, https://projectsemicolon.com.

15 Amy Bleuel, quoted in Gabrielle Olya, "Project Semicolon Empowers People Who Suffer from Depression," *People*, July 7, 2015, https://people.com/celebrity/project-semicolon-empowers-people-who-suffer-from-depression/.

4

COLONS AND DASHES

Purpose and Application

A colon formally introduces a list or other information that in some way further characterizes or expands upon the text that immediately precedes it. A colon can also introduce quotations, salutations, subtitles, and dialogue; and a colon can separate data. A colon can be followed by a word, series of words, phrase, independent clause, or several independent clauses (sentences). One space, **not** two, follows a colon.

A dash (also known as an *em* dash), which differs from a hyphen[1] and an *en* dash,[2] similarly allows for the expansion of ideas, but in different ways. Dashes can be used to emphasize parenthetical information, including abrupt changes in thought; complete the meaning of a sentence; introduce lists; and make certain punctuation-rich sentences easier to read. They can also show interrupted speech, format special cases of source attribution, and signify missing letters and words. Two dashes set off material that comes in the middle of a sentence (—*set-off text*—); a single dash sets off material that ends a sentence (—*set-off text*).

Colons

Introducing a List

4.1 Place a colon after an independent clause that introduces a list.

- My favorite forms of punctuation include the following: colons, dashes, and semicolons.
- These are my favorite forms of punctuation: colons, dashes, and semicolons.

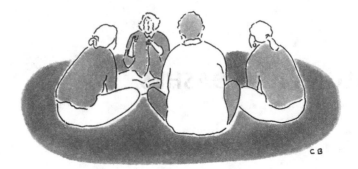

"And always remember that it is the gritty colon itself, not the half-baked semi-colon, that wields the power to confound even the most erudite minds."

Burke, Christopher; www.CartoonStock.com

4.2 Do **not** pause an otherwise fluid sentence by placing a colon after a verb or preposition (or a phrase like *such as*) that immediately precedes a list. In the examples below, **no** colon is needed after the italicized word(s).

INCORRECT My favorite forms of punctuation *include*: colons, dashes, and semicolons.

CORRECT My favorite forms of punctuation include colons, dashes, and semicolons.

INCORRECT My favorite forms of punctuation *include, for example*: colons, dashes, and semicolons.

CORRECT My favorite forms of punctuation include, for example, colons, dashes, and semicolons.

INCORRECT My favorite forms of punctuation *are*: colons, dashes, and semicolons.

CORRECT My favorite forms of punctuation are colons, dashes, and semicolons.

INCORRECT I have a full understanding *of*: colons, dashes, and semicolons.

CORRECT I have a full understanding of colons, dashes, and semicolons.

INCORRECT I use many forms of punctuation, *such as:* colons, dashes, and semicolons.

CORRECT I use many forms of punctuation, such as colons, dashes, and semicolons.

4.3 Use a colon to introduce a vertical list that takes the form of bulleted items, numbered or alphabetical items, or items presented in the form of narrative paragraphs ideally distinguished (set off) from the rest of the text.

Students will be tested tomorrow on three forms of punctuation:

- colons
- dashes
- semicolons

Students will be tested tomorrow on three forms of punctuation:

1. colons
2. dashes
3. semicolons

Students will be tested tomorrow on three forms of punctuation:

They will be expected to know how a colon can formally introduce a list or other information that in some way further characterizes or expands upon the text that immediately precedes it. Additionally, they'll need to know how a colon can also introduce quotations, salutations, subtitles, and dialogue; and how a colon can separate data.

They will be expected to know how dashes can be used to emphasize parenthetical information, including abrupt changes in thought; complete the meaning of a sentence; introduce lists; and make certain punctuation-rich sentences easier to read.

They will be expected to know that a semicolon connects closely related independent clauses and, conversely, separates items in a series having internal punctuation. And they will need to know how to recognize when a semicolon is incorrectly used in place of a comma.

In addition to being tested on three forms of punctuation (colons, dashes, and semicolons), students will be asked to . . .

RHETORICALLY SPEAKING

It is not uncommon, especially in more informal writing, to find a word or phrase (as opposed to an independent clause) introducing a list. The practice, though seldom addressed by style manuals or punctuation tutorials, is often embraced by skilled writers as a cogent, pointed way of introducing ideas.

- My three favorite punctuation marks used to be colons, dashes, and semicolons. My new favorites: ellipses and exclamation points.
- Our eating habits could not be more different. Him: hot dogs, hamburgers, and chili fries. Me: broccoli, carrots, and low-fat cottage cheese.

Similarly, an incomplete sentence followed by colon can effectively introduce a thought coming on the heels of another.

- He could lie, as he had done so many times before, to family, friends, and coworkers. Or: he could finally tell the truth.
- He had a couple of options. Choice one: tell the truth and let the chips fall where they may. Choice two: continue to misrepresent himself and forever live in fear of being discovered.

Introducing Supplemental Information

4.4 Place a colon after an independent clause when what follows either defines, explains, illustrates, summarizes, or elaborates upon elements in the clause.

- She got A's on the two most important tests: the midterm and the final. [defines]
- He believed he was the most popular kid in class for one reason only: he knew punctuation better than anyone in the fourth grade. [explains]
- They loved punctuation to this extreme: they actually named their two dogs Dash and Slash. [illustrates]
- They thought a period and comma were interchangeable and that a semicolon was a fancy name for a dash: clearly, they were punctuation challenged. [summarizes]
- Knowing how to use punctuation can profoundly impact your life: better grades, better jobs, and smarter dates await the punctuation perfect. [elaborates]

In cases where the second clause defines, explains, or illustrates the first, it is clear how a colon, as demonstrated above, works better than a semicolon. But when the second clause *summarizes* or *elaborates* upon the first clause, the difference between using a colon and a semicolon can sometimes be subtle, the choice between the two being more nuanced. In the last two examples above, a colon comes after the first independent clause because the second independent clause speaks more directly to the first. Still, a semicolon might *almost* have worked as well.

- They thought a period and comma were interchangeable and that a semicolon was a fancy name for a dash; clearly, they were punctuation challenged. [summarizes]
- Knowing how to use punctuation can profoundly impact your life; better grades, better jobs, and smarter dates await the punctuation perfect. [elaborates]

4.5 Style manuals differ on whether to capitalize the first word (other than a proper noun) of an independent clause that follows a colon. (*APA* and *AP Stylebook*, for instance, capitalize the first word; *Chicago*, *MLA*, and *Oxford Style* generally do **not**.[3]) It is common, though, to capitalize the first word when a colon introduces either a question; a declarative statement that normally would be capitalized (such as an adage, maxim, motto, principle, proverb, rule, or saying); or two or more sentences, regardless of whether they all are complete sentences.

- This was the most difficult question on the test: In what ways are colons and dashes alike?
- To increase membership, the campus Punctuation Club decided to adopt a new motto: Punctuation is our friend. Too, they agreed to be more considerate when correcting others' punctuation errors and to always follow the Golden Rule: Do unto others as you would have them do unto you.
- This is what they knew about writing: They were skilled in using correct punctuation and grammar. All the time. They could write unified and coherent paragraphs. All the time. And, they wrote with rhythm and grace. All the time.

4.6 Do **not** include more than one colon in a sentence.

INCORRECT She got A's on the two most important tests: the midterm and the final, and she aced her two other course assignments: the group project and personal journal.

CORRECT She got A's on the two most important tests: the midterm and the final, and she aced her two other course assignments, which were the group project and personal journal.

CORRECT She got A's on the two most important tests: the midterm and the final, and she aced her two other course assignments (the group project and personal journal).

CORRECT She got A's on the two most important tests: the midterm and the final, and she aced her two other course assignments—the group project and the personal journal.

Introducing Quotations, Salutations, Subtitles, and Dialogue

4.7 A colon can introduce a quotation (see Chapter 6: 6.3; 6.4; 6.5).

4.8 A colon follows a formal salutation (*Dear Professor Ortiz:*) (*To Whom It May Concern:*). In informal salutations, a comma suffices (*Dear Sunny,*). Sometimes a colon follows a name informally addressed without salutation (*Sunny:*).

4.9 A colon introduces the subtitle of a book or article.

- *Punctuation Revisited: A Strategic Guide for Academics, Wordsmiths, and Obsessive Perfectionists*
- "Style and the New Journalism: A Rhetorical Analysis of Tom Wolfe"

4.10 A colon introduces each speaker's words in traditionally formatted dialogue.

JAMAAL: Is this what you mean by using a colon to introduce my words?
WINONA: Yes, that's exactly what I mean.
JAMAAL: Thank you.
WINONA: You're welcome.

Separating Other Data

4.11 A colon separates data when expressing the time of day (6:30 p.m.); the minutes, hours, and seconds of a time period (2:31:16); ratios (4:1); Biblical references to chapter and verse (Psalm 23:4); memorandum headings (To: From: Date: Subject:); and when called for in reference citations (New York: Routledge).

RHETORICALLY SPEAKING

A sentence structured around a colon flags the attention of the reader because it promises more to come, but not before a staged pause (the colon) and a metaphorical drum roll. The colon is particularly effective for formally emphasizing bold statements and pointed questions.

- Asked whether he could ever be friends with someone who did not care about colons and dashes, his answer was unequivocal: No.
- The popular high school valedictorian dropped out of college, renounced Western culture, and moved to the Amazon. What her parents most wanted to know: Are you okay?

Dashes

Formatting Dashes

4.12 In the days of the typewriter, a dash (—)was formed by two consecutive hyphens (--) with **no** space before or after each hyphen. Today, computer word processing programs provide for dashes that reflect their true size, which is slightly longer than two consecutive hyphens, or approximately the width of a capital *M*. If you type two hyphens and leave **no** spaces between the words preceding and following the hyphens (*word--word*), most word processing programs will automatically convert the hyphens into an em dash. Dashes can also be accessed as a special character or symbol in most word processing programs.

4.13 A dash must appear on the same line as the word that immediately precedes it.

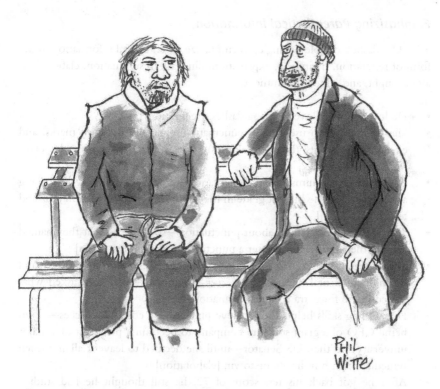

"I was a gainfully employed copy editor. Suddenly, one day, I couldn't tell an em dash from an en dash."

Witte, Phil; www.CartoonStock.com

INCORRECT Do not separate the dash from the word that precedes it
—got it?
CORRECT Do not separate the dash from the word that precedes it—got it?

AP STYLEBOOK

AP Stylebook places a space before and after the dash — as just demonstrated, "except [at] the start of sports agate summaries." *AP Stylebook* also clarifies the width of the dash: "An *em dash* is approximately the width of a capital letter *M* **in the typeface being used**" (emphasis added).[4] The smaller point sizes customary in newspapers (*The New York Times*, for example, uses 8.7 point Imperial typeface for its running text) and other venues account for why dashes appear in slightly varying—but proportional-to-text—lengths.

Emphasizing Parenthetical Information

4.14 Use dashes, double or single, to emphasize parenthetical information in the form of reiteration, definition, explanation, illustration, summation, elaboration, afterthought, and editorial comment.

- He loved—really loved—using dashes. [reiteration]
- She knew how to use ending punctuation—periods, question marks, and exclamation points (but not ellipses)—better than anyone in the class. [definition]
- He began to call himself Mr. Punctuation—a name inspired by his having always received the highest grade in the class on every punctuation quiz and test. [explanation]
- They relished everything about punctuation—so much so that they named each of their fourteen cats after a punctuation mark. [illustration]
- She missed the midterm examination, three quizzes, two group projects, and the individual oral presentation—*seven* assignments—and then asked what she could do for extra credit. [summation]
- Her writing skills helped her achieve phenomenal corporate success—from being CEO of a giant software company to becoming president of a major university and then US Senator—until she decided to leave it all and teach remedial English in her hometown. [elaboration]
- After he got back his test score of 72, he still thought he had studied effectively—or maybe not. [afterthought]
- He said he learned about punctuation when he was three—yeah, right. [editorial comment]

Sometimes parenthetical information takes the form of an abrupt change in thought.

- She would lie awake, wondering whether her third husband—or was it her fourth?—had ever learned the difference between a comma and a semicolon.
- I gathered my notes on punctuation at 7 a.m.—that is, assuming my new $8 watch was accurate—and studied right up until the test at noon.

RHETORICALLY SPEAKING

Parenthetical information can also be set off by commas, parentheses, or even explanatory footnotes (in cases where the information referenced is lengthy and less germane to the meaning of the sentence). Of these options, the dash provides the most dramatic, albeit informal, way of highlighting parenthetical information because it is so interruptive. Notice, for example, how *really loved* in the sample sentence below can be punctuated with increasing levels of emphasis.

- He loved (really loved) using dashes.
- He loved, really loved, using dashes.
- He loved—really loved—using dashes.

Thoughts set off by dashes, especially by double dashes, are arresting because the dash-text-dash structure briefly stops, starts, and stops the reader. Dashes provide more emphasis than do parentheses and commas.

Although material enclosed by parentheses is intended to be read with less emphasis than if it were enclosed by commas or dashes, a case can be made that parentheses, rather than being processed as mild asides, are actually more interruptive than commas, and, as such, unwittingly give more emphasis to the enclosed material than if it were set off by commas. The level of emphasis given to parenthetical material, however, is not just a matter of how much interruption occurs in the reading experience. Emphasis is also established by the reader's expectation of what it means when material is set off by parentheses as opposed to commas and dashes.

4.15 The information highlighted by a dash can be an independent clause appearing within the sentence.

- His writing became a punctuation-free zone—some called it a sanctuary where periods, commas, and the like never had to appear in public—that complemented his championing of syntactical anarchy.
- His writing became a punctuation-free zone—it was also a grammar-free zone—that complemented his championing of syntactical anarchy.

In these sentences, dashes do more than emphasize the set-off text. If **not** for dashes preceding and following the second independent clause in each sentence (*some called it a sanctuary where periods, commas, and the like never had to appear in public; it was also a grammar-free zone*), each sentence would have been a run-on, having fused two independent clauses. Parentheses can also set off an independent clause to aid readability, but the enclosed text would be emphasized less.

- His writing became a punctuation-free zone (some called it a sanctuary where periods, commas, and the like never had to appear in public) that complemented his championing of syntactical anarchy.
- His writing became a punctuation-free zone (it was also a grammar-free zone) that complemented his championing of syntactical anarchy.

4.16 An independent clause separated by dashes is usually neither capitalized nor followed by ending punctuation—unless the independent clause represents either a formal question; an exclamatory statement; or a declarative statement normally capitalized, such as an adage, maxim, motto, principle, proverb, rule, or saying. (*Oxford Style*, however, instructs otherwise: "Do not capitalize a word, other than a proper noun, after a dash, even if it begins a sentence."[5])

- The toughest question on the test—When would you use a colon versus a dash to introduce a list?—was answered correctly by most students.
- The professor embraced a simple, but zero-tolerance policy on plagiarism—Plagiarize a single word and you'll fail the course!—which everyone understood.
- The professor reminded students of an old proverb—The road to Hell is paved with good intentions—whenever anyone explained it was never his/her intention to misread the reader.

4.17 Dashes in the middle of a sentence come in pairs: the first dash that precedes the enclosed information must be coupled with a second dash that follows the enclosed information—unless the parenthetical comment that follows the dash completes an independent clause.

INCORRECT I like dogs—in particular, boxers and pitbulls, cats, rabbits, and turtles.
CORRECT I like dogs—in particular, boxers and pitbulls—cats, rabbits, and turtles.
CORRECT I like dogs—in particular, boxers and pitbulls; I also like cats, rabbits, and turtles.

4.18 Do **not** include more than one set of dashes in a sentence. A sentence with multiple dashes can create a disjointed text.

> After studying diligently all day—9 a.m. to 6 p.m.—we were well-prepared—or at least we thought we were prepared—to take the exam—but we were wrong.

Completing a Sentence's Meaning

4.19 Double dashes and single dashes can both highlight parenthetical information, but the single dash can also express and underscore elements central to the sentence's meaning. In the examples below, the information that follows the dash is essential (restrictive), **not** parenthetical; and it is also given greater emphasis because it ends the sentence.

- I felt sorry he had failed all his classes, lost his scholarship, and was placed on "conditional probation"—until I learned he had spent nearly the entire semester surfing in Puerto Rico.

- He will regain his scholarship—if he brings his GPA up to 2.0.
- Colons, semicolons, and dashes!—those varmints did me in at the National Punctuation Contest.
- Correct punctuation, grammar, usage, and, of course, my sense of 'being'—they invigorate my writing.

Introducing a List

4.20 A dash can introduce a list.

- She was a Chemistry major, which you would never have guessed by her favorite words—'deity', 'reality', and 'being'.
- She feared only three things—"Sunnyville's Punctuation Police," death, and taxes.

A dash and a colon can both introduce a list. But a dash, which is more informal than a colon, gives somewhat greater emphasis to the listed items because it is more dramatic in the sense of being more interruptive than a colon. As illustrated in 4.19, when a list is needed to complete the sentence's main thought, the list comes first, before the dash.

Avoiding Confusion

4.21 Use dashes (or parentheses, depending on the degree of emphasis desired) to set off material—often, but **not** always, in the form of an appositive with internal punctuation—that would be confusing if separated by commas.

ORIGINAL They continued to misuse certain punctuation marks, dashes, parentheses, and brackets, throughout their papers.

REVISION They continued to misuse certain punctuation marks—dashes, parentheses, and brackets—throughout their papers.

ORIGINAL No shortage of composition handbooks exists that treat, in addition to punctuation, grammar, usage, mechanics, and other topics.

REVISION No shortage of composition handbooks exists that treat—in addition to punctuation—grammar, usage, mechanics, and other topics.

Showing Interrupted Speech

4.22 Use a dash, **not** an ellipsis, to indicate interrupted speech.

INCORRECT Asa: "Here are the rules for using an ellipsis. First you need to ..."
Eva: "Enough! I know how to use an ellipsis."

CORRECT Asa: "Here are the rules for using an ellipsis. First you need to—"
Eva: "Enough! I know how to use an ellipsis."

Formatting Special Cases of Source Attribution

4.23 Use a dash before the source of an epigraph (a statement that heads the first page of a book, chapter, short story, or article, and is meant to convey the tenor of the work); do **not** place epigraphs in quotation marks (see Chapter 6: 6.18). Here, for example, are the epigraphs as they originally appeared, respectively, for Harper Lee's *To Kill a Mockingbird*,[6] Mario Puzo's *The Godfather*,[7] and Neil Gaiman's *Coraline*[8]:

Lawyers, I suppose, were once children.

—*Charles Lamb*

Behind every great fortune
there is a crime.

—Balzac

Fairy tales are more than true: not because
they tell us that dragons exist, but because
they tell us that dragons can be beaten.

—*G. K. Chesterton*

Note: The source of the epigraph and/or the epigraph itself can be italicized; however, this is a formatting decision and is **not** required.

4.24 Use a dash before the source of a quotation when formatted in such a way that the source separately follows the quotation, as shown in the King[9] and Truss[10] quotations below.

"I believe the road to hell is paved with adverbs, and I will shout it from the roof tops."

—*Stephen King*

"Are the colon and semicolon old-fashioned? No, but they are old."

—*Lynne Truss*

Signifying Missing Words or Letters

4.25 Use a 2-em dash (———) to indicate missing words or missing letters in a word, which come about because the word is unknown (somehow missing), or the word is being redacted because it is an expletive or needs to be kept confidential. A space comes before and after a 2-em dash signifying a missing word; **no** space comes before and after a 2-em dash signifying missing letters.

- Over and over, they tried to figure out what the tattered and torn treasure map meant to say when it told of gold under the big ——— and next to the small ———.

- Just because I occasionally misuse dashes and am not all that concerned about it was no reason for him to go all-ballistic and call me a dumb f——.
- Two administrators from the largest school district, Principal —— and Vice Principal —— agreed to testify confidentially before our task force investigating improprieties in standardized testing.

Omitting Preceding and Following Punctuation

4.26 Omit punctuation that would have preceded and followed the text had it been set off by parentheses or commas rather than dashes.

- Although the dash was a mark he loved (really loved), he sparingly used it.
  Or:
  Although the dash was a mark he loved—really loved—he sparingly used it.
- He loved, really loved, using dashes.
  Or:
  He loved—really loved—using dashes.

4.27 The following punctuation marks can immediately precede a dash:

- question mark (see 4.14, 4.16)
- exclamation point (see 4.16, 4.19)
- closing double quotation mark (see 4.19)
- closing single quotation mark (see 4.19)
- parenthesis (see 4.14)
- period, but only if it comes after an abbreviation (see 4.14, 4.18)

4.28 The following punctuation marks can immediately follow a dash:

- opening double quotation mark (see 4.20)
- opening single quotation mark (see 4.20)
- closing double quotation mark, but only if it is part of interrupted speech (see 4.22)

RHETORICALLY SPEAKING

The dash is more attention-grabbing—and more versatile—than any other form of punctuation. "The em dash," observes Karen Elizabeth Gordon in *The New Well-Tempered Sentence: A Punctuation Handbook for the Innocent, the Eager, and the Doomed,* "is much too energetic and impetuous to have its story put on hold: a streak, a comet flash, a leap across a gap, it's the most available of punctuation marks, just because its form and function sometimes seem the closest to the way we think and perceive relationships."[11] Is it any wonder that the dash is so popular, especially among accomplished writers? Still, when overused, it can result in halting sentences that impede coherent expression.

Notes

1 Among its multiple uses, a hyphen connects compound words (*long-term, sister-in-law, Garcia-Smith*), numbers (*twenty-one*), and fractions (*one-third*); compounds with prefixes or suffixes (ex-governor; governor-elect); words that together function as adjectives (*well-conditioned athlete, dog-friendly park, razor-thin laptop*); compounds formed when letters or numbers are combined with words (X-ray, 10-day diet); and words broken at the end of a line of text. Hyphens also separate Arabic numbers, such as telephone numbers (805-869-0235), social security numbers (599-42-6738), and any other separated series of numbers (such as credit card and invoice numbers) that do **not** represent a range. **No** space comes before or after a hyphen.

2 An en dash, broadly speaking, is the approximate width (–) of a lower-case *e*. An en dash is slightly longer than a hyphen and one-half as long as an em dash. En dashes generally function more like hyphens than em dashes in the sense they connect numbers and they connect words, with the en dash usually substituting for the word *to* or *through*. Use en dashes for numerical ranges (1:00–3:30 p.m.; 1995–2010; pages 10–15; a crowd of 500–600); incomplete numerical ranges (2016–); non-numerical ranges (Monday–Friday; June–September); scores (126–110; 21–7; 4–0); and various other types of word connections (Jones–Smith bill; Los Angeles–London flight). En dashes can be accessed as a special character or symbol in most word-processing programs (and by other ways). But because their input usually requires more effort than does a hyphen, many writers simply use hyphens in place of en dashes, leaving it to the printer, if one is involved, to make the appropriate changes. **No** space comes before or after an en dash, unless it is being used in place of a dash, as is the practice of some publications.

3 *APA*, 90; *AP Stylebook*, 322; *Chicago*, 392; *MLA*, 7th ed., 71; *Oxford Style*, 80.

4 *AP Stylebook*, 98.

5 *Oxford Style*, 87.

6 Harper Lee, *To Kill a Mockingbird* (New York: J. B. Lippincott & Co., 1960).

7 Mario Puzo, *The Godfather* (New York: G. P. Putnam's Sons, 1969).

8 Neil Gaiman, *Coraline*, illus. Dave McKean (New York: HarperCollins, 2002).

9 Stephen King, *On Writing: A Memoir of the Craft* (New York: Charles Scribner's Sons, 2000), 118.

10 Lynne Truss, *Eats, Shoots & Leaves: The Zero Tolerance Approach to Punctuation* (New York: Gotham Books, 2003), 111.

11 Karen Elizabeth Gordon, *The New Well-Tempered Sentence: A Punctuation Handbook for the Innocent, the Eager, and the Doomed*, rev. ed. (New York: Ticknor & Fields, 1993), 85.

5

APOSTROPHES

Purpose and Application

The two main purposes of an apostrophe are to indicate possession[1] and to represent the missing letter(s) in a contraction. Additionally, apostrophes signify what is missing when words and dates are expressed colloquially. And apostrophes can aid in the readability of certain plurals.

Indicating Possession

5.1 To form the possessive of a singular **common noun** (a noun that names a person, place, thing, activity, quality, or concept) or **indefinite pronoun** (a pronoun that names a nonspecific person or thing), add an apostrophe—or right, single quotation mark ('), **not** a left, single quotation mark (')—and an *s* (*'s*) after the last letter of the word.

Singular	Singular Possessive	Incorrect
boy	boy's (dog)	boys (dog); boys' (dog)
girl	girl's	girls; girls'
child	child's	childs; childs'
man	man's	mans; mans'
woman	woman's	womans; womans'
one	one's	ones; ones'
anyone	anyone's	anyones; anyones'
someone	someone's	someones; someones'
everyone	everyone's	everyones; everyones'
no one	no one's	no ones; no ones'
nobody	nobody's	nobodys; nobodys'

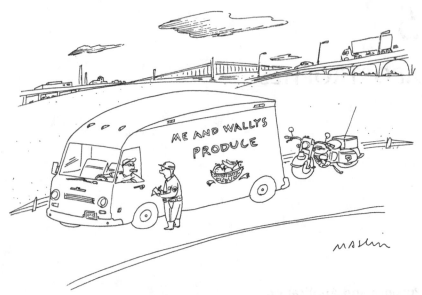

"Sorry, but I'm going to have to issue you a summons for reckless grammar and driving without an apostrophe."

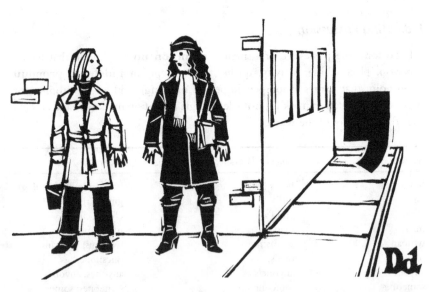

"My worst nightmare is seeing apostrophes where they don't belong."

5.2 To form the possessive of a plural noun ending in *s* or *es*, add an apostrophe after the *s* (*s'*) or *es* (*es'*).

Plural	Plural Possessive	Incorrect
boys	boys' (dog)	boys's (dog)
girls	girls'	girls's
Joneses	Joneses'	Joneses's

5.3 To form the possessive of an **irregular noun** (a noun made plural in a way other than by adding *s* or *es*), add an apostrophe and an *s* (*'s*).

Plural	Plural Possessive	Incorrect
children	children's	childrens; childrens'
men	men's	mens; mens'
women	women's	womens; womens'

5.4. To form the possessive of a singular common noun or a singular **proper noun** (a noun that begins with a capital letter and names a specific person, place, thing, activity, quality, or concept) ending in *s*, or ending in a letter sounding like *s* (*ce*, *x*, or *z*), add an *'s*.

> press's responsibility   Leon Uris's novel   Marion Jones's medals
> Rex's dog   Liz's cat   Mercedez's house   prince's castle

The conventional approach when forming the plural of singular nouns ending in *s* has been to let the sound of the construction govern decision-making and to **not** add *'s* if it hampers pronunciation. In particular, adding *'s* to words ending in *s* and having an *s* in their middle—such as *Jesus's*, *Moses's*, and *Demosthenes's*—can be phonetically challenging. But the trend is moving more towards adding the *'s* in these cases.

CHICAGO

Starting with its 16th edition, *Chicago* reversed two earlier positions. It "no longer recommends the traditional exception for proper classical names of two or more syllables that end in an *eez* sound." Whereas *Euripides' tragedies, the Ganges' source*, and *Xerxes' armies* was once the standard, now it is *Euripides's tragedies, the Ganges's source, Xerxes's armies*. And, "In a return to *Chicago*'s earlier practice, words and names ending in an unpronounced *s* form the possessive in the usual way (with the addition of an apostrophe and an *s*)." Instead of *Descartes' three dreams, the marquis' mother,* and *Francois' efforts, Chicago* now recommends *Descartes's three dreams, the marquis's mother, Francois's effort.*[2]

MLA, 7TH ED.

MLA advises, "To form the possessive of any singular proper noun, add an apostrophe and an *s*," even if the noun ends in *s*, as in "Venus's beauty" and "Dickens's reputation."[3]

APA

APA offers a brief discussion of possessive use consistent with *Chicago*, with this exception: "Use an apostrophe only with the singular form of names ending in unpronounced *s* (e.g., Descartes'). It is preferable to include *of* when referring to the plural form of names ending in unpronounced *s* (e.g., the home of the Descartes)."[4]

AP STYLEBOOK

AP Stylebook differs significantly from other style manuals when forming possessives. It requires adding only an apostrophe, **not** '*s*, to form the possessive of any singular *proper* noun ending in *s*: "Achilles' heel, Agnes' book, Ceres' rites, Descartes' theories, Dickens' novels, Euripedes' dramas, Hercules' labors, Jesus' life, Jules' seat, Kansas' schools, Moses' law, Socrates' life, Tennessee Williams' plays, Xerxes' armies." However, '*s* should be added to form the possessive of a singular *common* noun ending in *s*: "the hostess's invitation, the hostess's seat, the witness's answer, the witness's story." To form the possessive of a singular common or proper noun ending in a letter sounding like *s* (*ce, x,* or *z,*), add '*s*: "Butz's policies, the fox's den, the justice's verdict, Marx's theories, the prince's life, Xerox's profits."[5]

5.5 When two nouns share ownership, place the '*s* on the second noun. *Norman and Carmen's library contained hundreds of books on punctuation.* Or: *The library containing hundreds of books on punctuation was Norman and Carmen's.* If Norman and Carmen individually own libraries, both nouns would be possessive: *Norman's and Carmen's libraries* ... Or: *The libraries are Norman's and Carmen's.*

5.6 Possessive pronouns, such as *his, hers, its, ours, theirs, yours,* and *whose,* do **not** include apostrophes.

5.7 When you have a noun whose singular and plural forms both end in *s*— *economics, mathematics, politics, series, species,* for example—the singular and plural possessive are the same, both formed by adding an apostrophe after the *s.*

- The Department of Economics' student success was attributed to its peer mentoring program and its offering of several online economics' tutorial programs.
- Despite its marketing campaign, the new television series was similar to other television series in the sense that the series' storyline was much like many series' storylines.

CHICAGO

"The same rule applies when the name of a place or an organization or a publication (or the last element in the name) is a plural form ending in *s,* such as *the United States,* even though the entity is singular."[6] *The United States' policy supersedes Beverly Hills' policy.*

5.8 To form the possessive of a compound noun (nouns formed by two or more words), add *'s* to the last element in the compound noun.

sister-in-law's   secretary of state's   attorney general's
chief executive officer's   associate vice president's

To form the plural possessive of a compound noun, pluralize the first element and add *'s* to the last element in the construction.

sisters-in-law's   secretaries of state's   attorneys general's
chief executive officers'   associate vice presidents'

5.9 To form the possessive of a name comprised only of initials, add *'s* after the last initial.

FDR's New Deal   JFK's Inaugural Address   LBJ's experience   MLK's speeches

5.10 To form a double possessive (a construction where *of* precedes the possessive form), add *'s* or *s'* to the common or proper noun, depending on which is appropriate.

a friend of my brother's   a friend of my sister's   a friend of my parents'
a colleague of Sakile's   a colleague of James's   a colleague of the Joneses'

Note: What is possessed (i.e., what precedes the preposition *of*) in a double possessive reflects a category comprising more than one. *A colleague of Sakile's* implies that Sakile has more than one colleague. If Sakile has only one colleague, we would say, *the colleague of Sakile*, **not** *the colleague of Sakile's*, in the same way we say, *the mother of Sakile*, **not** *the mother of Sakile's*.

5.11 Do **not** use the double possessive form when (a) possession is **not** actually being represented, or (b) the noun or pronoun that follows *of* is inanimate.

- a student of Plato, *not* a student of Plato's★
- a critic of Marx, *not* a critic of Marx's
- a benefactor of the college, *not* a benefactor of the college's
- the owner of the house, *not* the owner of the house's

★*A student of Plato* is one who studies Plato. On the other hand, if Plato had personally taught the student (as he did Aristotle), it would be correct to refer to Aristotle as *a student of Plato's*.

RHETORICALLY SPEAKING

Double possessives are duplicative and often unnecessary, especially given most double possessives can be rewritten in more cogent ways. *Sakile's colleague*, for example, is more concise and direct than *a colleague of Sakile's*.

Sometimes both the possessive and double possessive can be ambiguous. A case in point: *My mom's painting* could refer to a painting *of* your mom, a painting *owned by* your mom, or a painting *done by* your mom. *A painting of my mom's* could refer to a painting *owned* or *done* by your mom. The meaning would be clearer if you were to say:

- The painting of my mom ...
- The painting owned by my mom ...
- The painting done my mom ...

5.12 A noun that precedes a **gerund** (a noun formed by adding *ing* to a verb, e.g., *walk* = verb; *walking* = gerund) may sometimes be possessive.

- Maria's walking improved her health.
- Mariusz's understanding of apostrophes was exceptional.
- It was the candidate's dancing that first caught the attention of the voters.

CHICAGO

"When the noun or pronoun follows a preposition [such as *about*, *for*, and *of* in the examples below], the possessive is usually optional," as in these *Chicago* examples:

- "She was worried about her daughter (*or* daughter's) going there alone."
- "I won't stand for him (*or* his) being denigrated."
- "The problem of authors (*or* authors') finding the right publisher can be solved."[7]

Adds Fowler: "The possessive with gerund may be on the retreat, but its use with proper names and personal nouns and pronouns persists in literary and formal writing. When the personal pronoun [such as *I, you, he, she, they*] stands in the initial position it looks certain that the possessive form will be preferred for a long time to come: e.g. *His being so capable was the only pleasant thing* ... ," as opposed to *Him being so capable* ...[8]

5.13 Use an *'s* when referencing generic academic degrees.

- I earned a bachelor's degree and a master's degree.
- I earned a bachelor's [*degree* is implied] and a master's [*degree* is implied].

When referencing specific academic degrees, it is customary to capitalize the degree (*Chicago*, however, does **not**) and to **not** include any apostrophes: *Associate of Arts/Associate of Arts degree, Bachelor of Arts/Bachelor of Arts degree, Bachelor of Science/Bachelor of Science degree, Bachelor of Arts in Communication, Bachelor of Science in Chemistry, Master of Arts/Master of Arts degree, Master of Science/Master of Science degree, Master of Arts in Communication, Master of Science in Chemistry, Master of Business Administration, Master of Public Administration, Master of Fine Arts.*

5.14 Certain expressions, although **not** quite expressing ownership, are treated as possessive: *a winter's day, one month's suspension, five weeks' vacation* (literally meaning: *a day of winter, a suspension of one month, five weeks of vacation*). Of course, one could also just as easily write: *a winter day, one-month suspension, five-week vacation.* "An apostrophe," *Oxford Style* notes, "is **not** used in adjectival constructions such as *three months pregnant.*"[9] Expressions such as *for appearance's sake* (meaning: for the sake of appearance) and *for convenience's sake* are treated as possessive constructions. So, too, are *for goodness' sake* and *for old times' sake*, although only an apostrophe follows the *s*.

> **AP STYLEBOOK**
>
> Only an apostrophe (**not** *'s*) should follow the last letter of a word ending in an *s* sound when that word is "followed by a word that begins with *s*: *for appearance' sake, for conscience' sake, for goodness' sake.* Use *'s* otherwise: *the appearance's cost, my conscience's voice.*"[10]

5.15 In highly informal writing, the possessive noun sometimes stands alone, the object of possession being implied.

- I'll meet you at Rafael's [house].
- It was mom's [necklace].
- Before ownership changed, it was the Ace Company's [property].

5.16 Do **not** place an apostrophe on an **attributive noun** (a noun that functions as an adjective to modify a noun).

> arms race   Boys Town   Firefighters Charitable Foundation
> Girls League   honors society   Veterans Day   Veterans Affairs

In these constructions, the first noun is attributive (modifying), **not** possessive; it functions as an adjective, rather than as a noun. *Boys Town*, for example, does **not** reference a town *owned* by boys; rather, it describes a town *for* boys. A plural irregular noun even when functioning as an attributive noun, however, should be treated as possessive.

> children's hospital   Santa Barbara Men's Golf Club   women's dormitory

Several holidays are conventionally expressed as singular possessive.

> Father's Day   Mother's Day   New Year's Day
> Saint Patrick's Day   Valentine's Day

(Parents' Day and Presidents' Day, on the other hand, are treated as plural possessive.)
    Style manuals and dictionaries sometimes disagree over what should be attributive versus possessive, as seen in the differences between *Chicago* and *AP Stylebook*.

> **CHICAGO**
>
> "Chicago dispenses with the apostrophe only in proper names (often corporate names) that do not officially include one. In a few established cases,

a singular noun can be used attributively; if in doubt, choose the plural possessive." *Chicago*'s examples: "children's rights (*or* child rights), farmers' market, women's soccer team, boys' clubs, veterans' organizations, players' unions, taxpayers' associations (*or* taxpayer associations), consumers' group (or consumer group)."[11]

AP STYLEBOOK

"Do not add an apostrophe to a word ending in *s* when it is used primarily in a descriptive sense: *citizens band radio, a Cincinnati Reds infielder, a teachers college, a Teamsters request, a writers guide.*"[12]

Determining whether a noun is attributive or possessive is further complicated by two factors:

First, some organizations/entities treat the first noun in their name as attributive, while other organizations/entities write it as possessive. Standard practice for style manuals and dictionaries is to follow the organization/entity's custom, irrespective of any collective consistency.

Actors' Equity   Barclays Bank   Barneys   Diners Club
Harrods   *Ladies' Home Journal*   Lands' End   Macy's   *Publishers Weekly*

(Barclays, Barney's, and Harrods now omit their possessive apostrophe, although they initially referenced family names: James Barclay, Barney Pressman, and Charles Henry Harrod.)

Second, the same noun can be attributive in one context and possessive in another depending on how it is used in the sentence, although here the differences are especially nuanced.

Wildcats quarterback [attributive] Dan Kaplan, who is probably the Wildcats' best quarterback [possessive] ever, embodies the Wildcats' winning-is-everything mindset [possessive], which he models at every Wildcats game [attributive] and notably during the Wildcats' ten-game winning streak [possessive].

5.17 Do **not** place parenthetical material immediately following a possessive noun.

INCORRECT The Modern Language Association's (MLA) position is …
INCORRECT The Modern Language Association's (MLA's) position is …

INCORRECT MLA's (The Modern Language Association) position is . . .
INCORRECT MLA's (The Modern Language Association's) position is . . .

Instead, revise the sentence to eliminate the possessive noun or the parenthetical information.

- The position of the Modern Language Association of America (MLA) is . . .
- The position of MLA (The Modern Language Association of America) is . . .
- The Modern Language Association's position is . . .
- MLA's position is . . .

5.18 Do **not** italicize the *'s* when forming the possessive of a normally italicized word, such as a title.

- *Twilight*'s popularity is owed to many factors.
- *The New Yorker*'s love of commas is legendary.

Note: The in-paragraph examples throughout this chapter, including examples with apostrophes, have been placed in all-italics solely for the purpose of distinguishing them within the text.

5.19 It is preferable to **not** put possessive words in quotation marks. Instead, revise the sentence to eliminate the possessive form. *The plot of "Rip Van Winkle,"* for example, is more legible than *"Rip Van Winkle"'s plot."*

RHETORICALLY SPEAKING

Purists will argue that inanimate objects cannot possess or own anything, and it is thus improper to speak, for example, of the *door's hinges, shirt's collar, hotel's lounge.* Instead, so goes the thinking, we should say the *hinges of the door, collar of the shirt, lounge in the hotel.* Another option, of course, would be to change the otherwise possessive noun into an attributive noun: *door hinges, shirt collar, hotel lounge.* Purists notwithstanding, most writers do not distinguish between animate and inanimate possession, except in the case of double possessives (see 5.11).

AP STYLEBOOK

"There is no blanket rule," *AP Stylebook* says, "against creating a possessive form for an inanimate object, particularly if the object is treated in a personified sense.... In general, however, avoid excessive personalization of inanimate objects, and give preference to an *of* construction when it fits the makeup of the sentence. For example, the earlier references to *mathematics' rules* and *measles' effects* would better be phrased: *the rules of mathematics, the effects of measles.*"[13]

Signifying Missing Letters and Numbers

5.20 Use an apostrophe to replace the missing letter(s) in a contraction.

can't   don't   haven't   I'll   I'm   it's   should've   there's
we'll   we're   weren't   who's   would've   you're

RHETORICALLY SPEAKING

Some contractions and possessive pronouns that sound alike are commonly confused. For example:

- *It's* serves as the contraction for *it is; its* is the possessive form of *it. It's* [it is] *the policy of the company to promote its best writers.* (There is no such construction as *its'.*) One way to test which form is correct is to replace *it's* or *its* with *it is.* If the sentence still makes sense, then use *it's;* if it does not, then use *its.* For example:

  1. *Its the company's policy to promote the best writers = It is the company's policy to promote the best writers.* Because the sentence makes sense with *it is, its* is incorrect and should be replaced with *it's.*

  2. *The company promotes it's best writers = The company promotes it is best writers.* Because the sentence does not make sense, *it's* is incorrect and must be replaced with *its.* This test can be applied as well to the examples below.

- *Who's* serves as the contraction for *who is; whose* is a possessive pronoun. *Any student who's* [who is] *majoring in English and whose career goal is to teach composition can apply for the scholarship.*
- *There's* serves as the contraction for *there is; theirs* is a possessive pronoun. *There's* [there is] *one thing of which I am certain: theirs was the best proposal.*
- *You're* serves as a contraction for *you are; your* is a possessive pronoun. *They thought your proposal was terrific, and you're* [you are] *the one they want to hire.*

5.21 In more colloquial venues, apostrophes can signify missing letters (in words) and missing numbers (in dates). *Nothin' happenin' 'cause I'm just hangin' and chillin', listening to rock 'n' roll, and trying to sound like I wasn't really born in '68, or was it '69?*

Avoiding Confusion

5.22 Use *'s* to form a plural when adding *s* alone might be confusing, such as when pluralizing letters. The use of apostrophes in the second example prevents the reader from confusing *a's*, *b's*, and *i's* with *as*, *bs*, and *is*.

INCORRECT She used to get bs in all her classes. Now it is as, except for the two is she received when she dropped out of school to attend Punctuation Rehab.

CORRECT She used to get b's in all her classes. Now, it is a's, except for the two i's she received when she dropped out of school to attend Punctuation Rehab.

Better yet, use capital letters to enhance legibility when representing academic grades.

> She used to get B's in all her classes. Now, it is A's, except for the two I's she received when she dropped out of school to attend Punctuation Rehab.

MLA, 7TH ED.

MLA suggests adding *'s* when pluralizing any letter, whether lower-case or upper-case.[14] Most style manuals, however, call for the use of *'s* only with lower case letters, which are less legible without benefit of *'s*.

5.23 The trend is away from using *'s* to form plurals of letter abbreviations and more toward adding just *s*: *BAs, PhDs, CDs, CVs, PCs, CPUs, URLs*. The plurals of dates, numbers, and numbers expressed as words follow suit: *1970s, two 5s, four threes*. Similarly, to form the plural of words referenced as words, add *s* or *es* with **no** apostrophe: *ands, buts, ifs, maybes, nos, whys, yeses*. Other dos and don'ts: If you italicize a pluralized word in normal exposition (as opposed to the examples above that have been placed in all–italics to distinguish them from the rest of the text), do **not** italicize the *s*: *and*s, *but*s, *if*s, *maybe*s, *no*s, *why*s, *yes*es.

RHETORICALLY SPEAKING

Glaring apostrophe mistakes, which many readers can easily spot, can swiftly diminish your credibility. Such errors include omitting the necessary apostrophe before the s—*childs* toy, *anyones* guess, *womens* department, *mens* clothes—or the needed apostrophe after the s: the three *classmates* project. Equally cringeworthy is the incorrect use of apostrophes to form plurals, often called *greengrocer's apostrophes*, a reference to British grocers who were called "greengrocers" because they sold fruit and vegetables in small shops and whose product for-sale signs used apostrophes in forming plurals, such as *apple's, orange's, carrot's, potatoe's*. Knowing at least the basic rules of apostrophe use can prevent these kinds of errors.

Those lacking confidence in their punctuation skills tend to rely heavily, if not solely, on grammar/punctuation computer checkers, faithfully following every suggestion even when the counsel includes adding unnecessary apostrophes or foregoing necessary ones. Grammar/ punctuation computer checkers are helpful aids, not decrees, whose advice functions best when critically assessed by the knowledgeable writer.

APOSTROPHES: KEY DIFFERENCES BETWEEN AMERICAN AND BRITISH STYLE

❖   In contrast to *Chicago*, *Oxford Style* recommends, "With singular nouns that end in an *s* sound, the extra *s* can be omitted if it makes the phrase difficult to pronounce (*the catharsis' effects*), but it is often preferable to transpose the words and insert *of* (*the effects of the catharsis*)."[15]

❖   *Oxford Style* also embraces the common practice (again, with the exception of *Chicago*) of including "an apostrophe alone after classical names ending in *s* or *es*," such as *Euripides'*, although it is acceptable, *Oxford Style* says, to use *'s* with shorter names, such as *Zeus's*.[16]

Notes

1   Also known as genitive case, possessive case describes different kinds of semantic relationships (as discussed throughout this chapter), with "true possession, as ordinarily understood, being only one" *Chicago*, 231.

2   University of Chicago Press, *The Chicago Manual of Style*, 16th ed. (Chicago: University of Chicago Press, 2010), 354.

3   *MLA*, 7th ed., 75.

4   *APA*, 97.

5 *AP Stylebook*, 227–28.
6 *Chicago*, 423.
7 *Chicago*, 426.
8 Butterfield, ed., *Fowler's Dictionary of Modern English Usage*, 640.
9 *Oxford Style*, 70.
10 *AP Stylebook*, 228.
11 *Chicago*, 425.
12 *AP Stylebook*, 228.
13 *AP Stylebook*, 321.
14 *MLA*, 7th ed., 74.
15 *Oxford Style*, 69.
16 *Oxford Style*, 71.

6

DOUBLE AND SINGLE QUOTATION MARKS

Purpose and Application

Double quotation marks and single quotation marks indicate which words are those of another speaker or writer. Quotation marks are also used to indicate the titles of various works and to call attention to certain words and phrases.

Double Quotation Marks

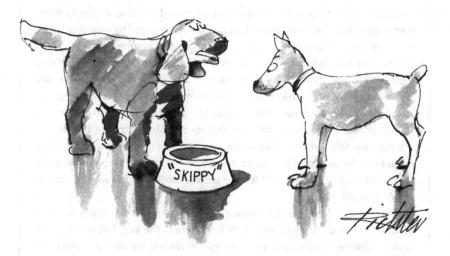

"I insisted on the quotation marks."

Quoting Others

6.1 Use quotation marks to indicate you are quoting the words of others.

> Sylvia Plath said: "And by the way, everything in life is writable about if you have the guts to do it, and the imagination to improvise. The worst enemy to creativity is self-doubt."[1]

The source, *Sylvia Plath*, can also appear after, as well as in the middle, of the quotation. When the source comes in the middle, the quotation marks must stop and start around the interjection of the source.

- "And by the way, everything in life is writable about if you have the guts to do it, and the imagination to improvise. The worst enemy to creativity is self-doubt," said Sylvia Plath.
- "And by the way, everything in life is writable about if you have the guts to do it, and the imagination to improvise," said Sylvia Plath. "The worst enemy to creativity is self-doubt."
- "And by the way, everything in life is writable about if you have the guts to do it, and the imagination to improvise. The worst enemy to creativity," said Sylvia Plath, "is self-doubt."

RHETORICALLY SPEAKING

Deciding where to provide source attribution and whether it should interrupt a quotation presents more than just an opportunity to vary your style. It also allows you to communicate subtle degrees of emphasis.

The first example above (attribution followed by full quotation: *Sylvia Plath said ...*) positions the author ahead of the quotation. In contrast, the first bulleted example that follows (full quotation followed by attribution) elevates the quotation over the author. The second bulleted example uses source attribution between the two sentences to briefly pause the reader, allowing the first sentence (*And by the way, everything in life is writable about if you have the guts to do it, and the imagination to improvise*) to momentarily stand alone, an "opening act" for the second sentence (*The worst enemy to creativity is self-doubt*).

The third bulleted sample highlights the first sentence, which is introduced without attribution, and then underscores the key, last word in the second sentence (*self-doubt*) by pausing the reader, via source attribution, midway through the sentence.

Introducing Quotations

6.2 When an incomplete sentence—usually in the form of *he/she said* or some other variation of source attribution along with a verb, such as *asked, confessed, declared, exclaimed, noted, observed, proclaimed, stated, wrote*—informally introduces a quotation, a comma follows the attribution.

- Plath wrote, "The worst enemy to creativity is self-doubt."
- Plath observed, "The worst enemy to creativity is self-doubt."

When source attribution follows a quotation, the comma comes before the attribution.

- "The worst enemy to creativity is self-doubt," Plath wrote.
- "The worst enemy to creativity is self-doubt," observed Plath.

However, if the quotation or the quoted/italicized title ends with a question mark or exclamation point, **no** comma follows the mark or the point—*unless* the mark or point is part of a title *and* is followed by material normally set off by commas.

- "Is it snowing?" Antoinette asked.
- "It is snowing!" Antoinette exclaimed.
- "My favorite play is *Who's Afraid of Virginia Woolf?*" he said.
- "My favorite play is *Who's Afraid of Virginia Woolf?*, Edward Albee's critically acclaimed story about marital discord, which was later made into a popular film," he said.
- "I just read *The Sense of Style: The Thinking Person's Guide to Writing in the 21st Century!*" she said.
- "I just read *The Sense of Style: The Thinking Person's Guide to Writing in the 21st Century!*, Steven Pinker's insightful book on how to write in a clear and coherent style," she said.
- "Are you familiar with 'Where Do You Get Your Ideas?,' an essay by Neil Gaiman, the author of the comic book series *The Sandman*?" asked the professor. [The question mark after *Sandman* is **not** italicized because it is **not** part of the title.]

6.3 A colon, instead of comma, can be used after an incomplete introductory sentence to emphasize or dramatize the quotation that follows.

- The teacher warned: "No cheating."
- The jury concluded: "All are guilty."

6.4 When a complete sentence formally introduces a quotation, a colon follows the introduction.

- Sylvia Plath recognizes the major obstacle many writers face: "The worst enemy to creativity is self-doubt."
- Many well-known writers, such as Gustav Flaubert, are critical of their own work and how it falls short of their expectations: "It's as if a man with a good ear played his violin out of tune; his fingers just refuse to produce the right sound although that sound is in his head."[2]

6.5 When a complete or incomplete sentence introduces a quotation comprising two or more sentences, a colon follows the introduction.

6.6 When you introduce a quotation by integrating it with your own words to form a seamless construction, punctuate the sentence just as you would normally; do **not** insert any additional commas that you would **not** otherwise include if the quoted material were **not** in quotation marks.

INCORRECT I have been told that, "double and single quotation marks are not difficult to master."
CORRECT I have been told that "double and single quotation marks are not difficult to master."
INCORRECT I have been told that "most punctuation marks are easy to learn," if you set your mind to it.
CORRECT I have been told that "most punctuation marks are easy to learn" if you set your mind to it.

6.7 When starting a quotation, it is generally acceptable to change the first word to upper or lower case to fit the syntax of your sentence. If your professor says, *Fortunately, most punctuation marks are easy to learn; moreover, most punctuation marks are fun to use*, you could write:

- My professor says that "fortunately, most punctuation marks are easy to learn."
- My professor contends, "Most punctuation marks are fun to use."

6.8 When textual precision is mandated by special contexts, such as a legal document, or is otherwise required by a particular style manual, indicate changes in capitalization by bracketing the first letter of the word you changed. Had the preceding examples qualified, they would have taken this form:

- My professor says that "[f]ortunately, most punctuation marks are easy to learn."
- My professor contends, "[M]ost punctuation marks are fun to use."

Introducing Block Quotations

6.9 Longer quotations should be separated from the body of your text and formatted as an indented block of type without quotation marks. This holds true for
longer quotations from speeches, lectures, plays, and media (such as film, television,
and sound recordings), which should also be blocked. In a block quotation, use
double quotation marks to indicate when the quotation includes quotations from
other sources or other types of material normally placed in quotation marks.

Style manuals differ somewhat about when the length of quoted material
requires blocking. *MLA*, for example, says to set off quotations of "more
than four lines when run into the text."³ *APA* requires they be 40 words or
longer,⁴ while *Chicago* opts for 100 words or more, or when the quotation
is two or more paragraphs long, or in special circumstances, such as quoted
correspondence that includes salutations and signatures.⁵ *Oxford Style*, on the
other hand, blocks quotations of 50 or more words.⁶ Because they almost
always run more than two sentences, block quotations are usually introduced
with a colon. Footnotes or in-text citations normally come at the end of a
block quotation.

In *Simple and Direct: A Rhetoric for Writers*, Jacques Barzun writes:

> A good judge of the facts has declared: "All writing is rewriting." He
> meant good writing, for easy reading. The path to rewriting is obvi-
> ous: when reading after a shorter or longer lapse of time what one
> has written, one feels dissatisfaction with this or that word, sentence,
> paragraph—or possibly with the whole effort, the essay or chapter....
> If words you have set down puzzle you once you have forgotten how
> they came to your mind, they will puzzle the stranger and you must
> do something about them—rediscover your meaning and express *it*,
> not some other or none at all.⁷

In *Simple and Direct: A Rhetoric for Writers,* Jacques Barzun writes:

> A good judge of the facts has declared: "All writing is rewriting." He
> meant good writing, for easy reading. The path to rewriting is obvi-
> ous: when reading after a shorter or longer lapse of time what one
> has written, one feels dissatisfaction with this or that word, sentence,
> paragraph—or possibly with the whole effort, the essay or chapter....
> If words you have set down puzzle you once you have forgotten how
> they came to your mind, they will puzzle the stranger and you must do
> something about them—rediscover your meaning and express *it*, not
> some other or none at all. (Barzun 1975, 183)

[In a block quotation, as shown here, the in-text citation is positioned
separately from the last sentence.]

Note: The minimum length requirements for blocking poetry differ slightly from those of prose. *MLA*: "Verse quotations of more than three lines should be set off from your text as a block."[8] *Chicago*: block verse quotations of "two or more lines," unless the verse appears in a note, in which case "three or more" lines of quoted verse should be blocked.[9]

> In her poem, "A Word Is Dead," Emily Dickinson contrasts one view of language to that of her own.

> A word is dead
> When it is said,
> Some say.
> I say it just
> Begins to live
> That day.[10]

6.10 Block quotations can be introduced with a period-ending sentence if the sentence and the block quotation form a fluid narrative.

> In *Simple and Direct: A Rhetoric for Writers,* Jacques Barzun explores the importance of rewriting and the process it entails.

> > A good judge of the facts has declared: "All writing is rewriting." He meant good writing, for easy reading. . . .

> Quotation marks, Keith Houston reminds us, aren't exactly the flashiest form of punctuation.

> > For the most part these acrobatic commas glide along serenely under the radar, marking out dialogue, signaling an ironic "scare quote," or signposting unfamiliar "terminology." They are paragons of unshowy functionality. . . .[11]

6.11 In block quotations of one paragraph or less, the first line is **not** indented. Quotations of two or more paragraphs should match the paragraphing of the original text; the first paragraph of a multi-paragraph block quotation, however, should **not** be indented.

6.12 Should you face formatting constraints or specific editorial guidelines that preclude the blocking of quotations and instead mandate they be integrated into the text, as required by *AP Stylebook*, place quotation marks at the start of each new paragraph, but assign a closing quotation mark only after the last word of the final quoted paragraph.[12]

Quoting Dialogue

6.13 When you create dialogue or report on dialogue you have observed, begin a new paragraph every time the dialogue shifts to a new speaker, regardless of whether the speaker's name accompanies the quoted words. This allows the reader to follow along more easily.

> "I dreamed of someday having an argument with you *and winning*," she said.
> "That's happened. You've won sometimes," he said.
> "No, I haven't."
> "Yes, you have."
> "No."
> "Yes."
> "No. You're too good. Always so logical, so prepared, so focused."
> "Ok, maybe I am. Maybe ..."
> "Just say it."
> "Ok, you've never won an argument with me!"
> "Until now."

6.14 When you quote dialogue from another source (such as from a book, play, film, or television production), block the dialogue. Identify each speaker but do **not** place their words in quotation marks.

> Among the many classic scenes from the film *Casablanca* is when the protagonist, American expatriate Rick Blaine, who owns Rick's Café Americain, is being quizzed by Captain Louis Renault, the Chief of Police.
>
> > LOUIS RENAULT: And what in heaven's name brought you to Casablanca?
> > RICK BLAINE: My health. I came to Casablanca for the waters.
> > LOUIS RENAULT: The waters? What waters? We're in the desert!
> > RICK BLAINE: I was misinformed.[13]

Positioning Commas and Periods within Quotations

6.15 Place periods and commas—even if they are **not** part of the original quotation—inside (or before) the closing quotation mark. This holds true even if just one word is quoted (see Chapter 1: 1.12).[14]

INCORRECT Kellie never dated anyone who didn't first pass her two-hour punctuation test, which she simply referred to as "preconditions".
CORRECT Kellie never dated anyone who didn't first pass her two-hour punctuation test, which she simply referred to as "preconditions."

INCORRECT Her friends thought it was all a bit "wacko", but they still supported her.

CORRECT Her friends thought it was all a bit "wacko," but they still supported her.

Semicolons and colons, however, should be placed outside (or after) the quotation mark, unless they are part of the original quotation. (For more on how to position periods, question marks, and exclamation points with quoted material, see Chapter 1.)

Paraphrasing Quotations

6.16 When you paraphrase someone else's writing, you must rewrite it principally in your own words; it is **not** sufficient to change just a few lines here and there. Quotation marks must identify those words in your paraphrase, if any, that remain identical to the original. You must also cite the source that inspired your paraphrase. Here is how you might mostly paraphrase Barzun:

> In *Simple and Direct: A Rhetoric for Writers*, Jacques Barzun contends that writing is basically the act of rewriting. To create a well-written piece that is easy to read, Barzun maintains, you have to let your writing set for a while. After you pick it up again, you will sense "dissatisfaction with this or that word, sentence, paragraph" and know it needs to be changed. When you are unsure what your writing means because you cannot recall what you originally intended to say, imagine how it will "puzzle the stranger" reading your words for the first time.

Placing Other Works in Quotation Marks

6.17 Place double quotation marks around the titles of articles, essays, and opinion pieces appearing in journals, magazines, and newspapers; book chapters; short stories; poems (unless they are book length); unpublished works (for example, dissertations, theses, academic papers/presentations); nursery rhymes; fairy tales and fables; songs; blog posts, and specific episodes of television series, radio programs, and podcasts. (Style manuals sometimes differ on how to punctuate reference and bibliographic citations. *APA*, for example, does **not** place article titles in quotation marks.[15]) Again, commas and periods go inside the ending quotation marks.

> My favorite *Seinfeld* episodes include "The Contest," "The Puffy Shirt," and the "Parking Garage."

Italicize (do **not** place in quotation marks) titles of books, films, plays, operas, pamphlets, reports, journals, magazines, newspapers, (recurring) cartoons and comic strips, art work (such as paintings, drawings, lithographs, photographs), video games, record albums, blogs, television series, radio programs, and podcasts.

AP STYLEBOOK

"AP does not italicize words in news stories."[16] All titles otherwise italicized should be placed in quotation marks.[17]

6.18 Do **not** place epigraphs in quotation marks. The way an epigraph is uniquely formatted—usually set in a different font, positioned at the top of the page, and followed immediately by its author—indicates it is a quotation. Below, for example, is the epigraph from Ray Bradbury's *Fahrenheit 451*[18] (for additional examples of epigraphs, see Chapter 4: 4.23):

> If they give you ruled paper, write the other way.
>
> —*Juan Ramón Jiménez*

Calling Attention to Specific Words

6.19 Quotation marks can be employed in lieu of italics to call attention to specific words referenced or defined within a sentence.

- People use the word *grammar* to refer to a slew of writing problems, some of which deal with *usage*.

  Or:

- People use the word "grammar" to refer to a slew of writing problems, some of which deal with "usage."

6.20 Writers will sometimes place quotation marks around selected words as a way of negatively editorializing.

> Some "experts" downplay the importance of punctuation and insist that beginning writers need to learn "more important" things.

Quotation marks in this context, known as *scare quotes*, are meant to suggest the same disdain one conveys when using air quotes. These mocking tactics can be interpreted as petty and should be used prudently.

6.21 With few exceptions, do **not** use single quotation marks to highlight single words or phrases; instead, use double quotation marks, as shown above, or italics.

One exception: Use single quotation marks when following the unique conventions of a specific discipline, such as philosophy, theology, and linguistics, where certain words have specialized meanings. Philosophers writing within their discipline, for example, will speak of 'deity', 'reality', and 'being'. Here, the single quotation mark is considered part of the word; hence, commas and periods come after, **not** before, the single quotation mark (see Chapter 1: 1.13).

- Punctuation is the essence of my 'being'.
- My yoga instructor said, "Punctuation is the essence, or 'reality', of my 'being'."

A second exception: Place cultivars (plants cultivated through selective breeding) in single quotation marks. For example: 'Mister Lincoln' (rose), 'Himrod' (grape), and 'Yabukita' (tea).

RHETORICALLY SPEAKING

Writers sometimes make the mistake of over-quoting when it would have been more economical and on point to quote less and paraphrase more. Because readers assign greater importance to quoted text, extended quotations are best reserved for when they stylistically express your point more cogently and more elegantly than any possible paraphrase.

Single Quotation Marks

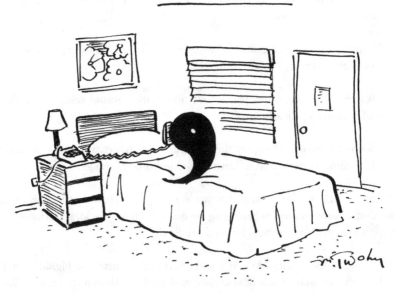

"Miss you, too."

Mike Twohy/The New Yorker Collection/The Cartoon Bank; Condé Nast

Quoting within a Quotation

6.22 Use single quotation marks when your quoted material includes quotations from other sources, titles typically placed in quotation marks (see 6.17), or specialized words called out by quotation marks, as shown above. Place periods and commas inside (or before) the closing single quotation mark.

- Don Watson, author of *Death Sentences: How Clichés, Weasel Words, and Management-Speak Are Strangling Public Language*, writes: "Martin Amis might be right. 'The professionalization of ordinary existence: this is the enemy within.' Language, after all, defines ordinary existence. 'Speak, that I may see thee.' It's how we know each other."[19]
- In *Expletive Deleted: A Good Look at Bad Language*, Ruth Wajnryb says: "There are two potential points of confusion when it comes to understanding and talking about foul language. One has to do with the words used that commonly *constitute* 'swearing.' The other has to do with how we *refer* to 'swearing.'"[20]
- Constance Hale comments on the royal *we* in *Sin and Syntax: How to Craft Wickedly Effective Prose*: "Editors also use the royal *we* (calling it 'the editorial *we*'). Remember all those 'Talk of the Town' pieces in the pre-Tina *New Yorker*? Lesser mortals—and writers not yet in *New Yorker* nirvana—might want to heed Mark Twain's advice, 'Only presidents, editors, and people with tapeworms ought to have the right to use *we*.'"[21]

As noted in Chapter 1 (1.14), legibility can be enhanced by including a slight space between single and double quotation marks when positioned together: (' "), rather than ('").

6.23 If your quoted material includes a quotation within a quotation, place double quotation marks around the innermost quotation.

> Jessica revealed, "My friend Ariel always tells her class, 'I love punctuation because it is one more way of applying, as Aristotle would say, "all the available means of persuasion," which every writer and speaker should want to do.'"

The convention is to start with double quotation marks and then alternate between single and double marks for each new quotation appearing within the original. This holds true for block quotations as well.

AP STYLEBOOK

Use single quotation marks when writing newspaper headlines.[22]

- Michelle Obama's Memoir 'Becoming' Breaks Sales Records
- Study Concludes Punctuation-Proficient Students 'Happier and Healthier'

QUOTATION MARKS: KEY DIFFERENCES BETWEEN AMERICAN AND BRITISH STYLE

British usage of quotation marks (what the British call *inverted commas*) differs significantly from American usage. *Oxford Style* recommends:

❖   Enclose quoted material in single, **not** double, quotation marks. Opposite to American custom, British practice begins with single quotation marks and then alternates between double and single marks for each new quotation appearing within the original. British newspapers, though, usually reverse the style and follow American practice.[23]

❖   Use single quotation marks to call out specific words and phrases.[24]

❖   Generally, place commas (unless they are part of the quotation) and periods outside of single and double quotation marks. If, however, the quoted material represents a grammatically complete sentence, place the period inside the closing quotation mark.[25] Compare, for example, these two sentences:

•   In *Digital Shift: The Cultural Logic of Punctuation*, Jeff Scheible observes, 'It is important to understand, then, that punctuation's history coincides closely with the history of the mechanical reproduction of written language.'[26] [The quoted material forms a complete sentence.]

•   Jeff Scheible observes that the history of punctuation 'coincides closely with the history of the mechanical reproduction of written language'. [The quoted material does **not** form a complete sentence.]

Notes

1 Sylvia Plath, *The Journals of Sylvia Plath*, eds. Ted Hughes and Francis McCollough (New York: Anchor Books, 1998), 85.
2 Gustav Flaubert, quoted in Rosemary Lloyd, "Flaubert's Correspondence," in *The Cambridge Companion to Flaubert*, ed. Timothy Unwin (Cambridge: Cambridge University Press, 2004), 75.
3 *MLA*, 8th ed., 76.
4 *APA*, 92.
5 *Chicago*, 711–12.
6 *Oxford Style*, 160.
7 Jacques Barzun, *Simple & Direct: A Rhetoric of Writers* (New York: Harper & Row, 1975), 183.
8 *MLA*, 8th ed., 78.
9 *Chicago*, 719; see also 761.

10 *The Poems of Emily Dickinson*, ed. Thomas H. Johnson (Cambridge, MA: The Belknap Press of Harvard University Press, 1955), 845.

11 Keith Houston, *Shady Characters: The Secret Life of Punctuation, Symbols & Other Typographical Marks* (New York: W.W. Norton & Company, 2013), 187.

12 *AP Stylebook*, 328.

13 *Casablanca*. Directed by Michael Curtiz. Los Angeles: Warner Brothers, 1942.

14 Periods, as discussed in Chapter 1, go inside (or before) the ending quotation mark, unless parenthetical material follows the quotation.

15 *APA*, 198–202.

16 *AP Stylebook*, 156.

17 *AP Stylebook*, 63–64.

18 Ray Bradbury, *Fahrenheit 451* (New York: Ballantine Books, 1953).

19 Don Watson, *Death Sentences: How Clichés, Weasel Words, and Management-Speak Are Strangling Public Language* (New York: Gotham Books, 2005), xxi.

20 Ruth Wajnryb, *Expletive Deleted: A Good Look at Bad Language* (New York: Free Press, 2005), 15.

21 Constance Hale, *Sin and Syntax: How to Craft Wickedly Effective Prose* (New York: Broadway Books, 1999), 46.

22 *AP Stylebook*, 134.

23 *Oxford Style*, 92, 162–63.

24 *Oxford Style*, 92–93.

25 *Oxford Style*, 163–64. For additional discussion of British guidelines on the use of quotation marks, see *Oxford Style*, 92–93, 160–64.

26 Jeff Scheible, *Digital Shift: The Cultural Logic of Punctuation* (Minneapolis: University of Minnesota Press, 2015), 10.

7

ELLIPSES AND SLASHES

Purpose and Application

The ellipsis (plural = *ellipses*) serves as an editorial tool and a literary device. The purpose of an *editorial* ellipsis is to indicate when you are omitting one or more words from a quotation. An ellipsis allows you to capture that portion of the original quotation that directly speaks to your editorial aim. Omitting less important text also saves space and moves the reader more quickly to your point. Ellipses are especially handy in academic writing, where you must often rely upon quoted material from primary texts and secondary sources to build and bolster your arguments. The purpose of a *literary* ellipsis, on the other hand, is to indicate theatrical pause, reflection, incomplete thought, and halting expression.

Designed to save space, the slash (/), which is also referred to as a *forward slash*, *solidus*, *stroke*, or *virgule*, functions in two opposite ways: it can provide a choice between paired words or, it can unite paired words. Additionally, slashes can separate lines of poetry, as well as serve to abbreviate and format certain types of information. The backward slash (\) is a typographical mark or symbol; it is **not** a form of punctuation.

Ellipses

Formatting Ellipses

7.1 Although some style manuals differ in their formatting of ellipses, the most common practice, which also achieves the greatest degree of legibility, is to use three consecutive points represented by period marks (. . .), with one space between each point, and one space before and after the ellipsis. (In the examples

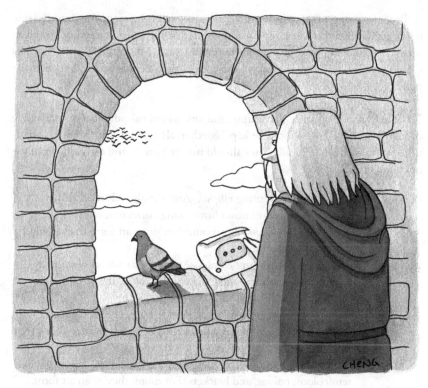

Alice Cheng/The New Yorker Collection/The Cartoon Bank; Condé Nast

below and many that follow, quotation marks have been added—even in what would otherwise be a block quotation—to illustrate how they would align with ellipses and parentheses.)

ORIGINAL   "My mom really, truly, surely loves using ellipses."
INCORRECT "My mom...surely loves using ellipses."
INCORRECT "My mom... surely loves using ellipses."
INCORRECT "My mom ...surely loves using ellipses."
INCORRECT "My mom...surely loves using ellipses."
CORRECT   "My mom ... surely loves using ellipses."

AP STYLEBOOK

An ellipsis is formatted with **no** spaces between points, and one space before and after the ellipsis.[1] *"My mom ... surely loves using ellipses."*

Proper spacing of an ellipsis usually requires that it be manually inputted one point at a time, rather than copied and inserted in the form of a symbol or character, as found in word processing programs, such Microsoft Word's "Special Characters," where the ellipsis provided does **not** include spaces between the points.

7.2 The points comprising an ellipsis and any additional punctuation preceding or following the ellipsis should be kept together, along with concluding punctuation, on the same line; ideally, they should **not** be broken and carried over to the next line of the page.

ORIGINAL   "My mom loves using ellipses. And she also adores commas (which she always knows how to use correctly), semicolons, colons, and brackets. For mom, they're an art form that should be practiced all the time."

INCORRECT "My mom loves using ellipses. And she also adores commas . . . , semicolons, colons, and brackets. For mom, they're an art form. . . ."

INCORRECT "My mom loves using ellipses. And she also adores commas. . ., semicolons, colons, and brackets. For mom, they're an art form . . . ."

CORRECT   "My mom loves using ellipses. And she also adores commas . . . , semicolons, colons, and brackets. For mom, they're an art form. . . ."

When a quotation mark follows an ellipsis, **no** space comes between the end of the ellipsis and the quotation mark.

INCORRECT "For my mom, punctuation is an art form. . . . "
CORRECT "For my mom, punctuation is an art form. . . ."

Omitting Text

7.3 Generally, when you omit text from a quoted passage, you must insert an ellipsis where the text ordinarily would have gone.

ORIGINAL "My mom really, truly, surely loves using ellipses. She uses ellipses all the time, and I do mean all the time, because she appreciates their function."

EDITED "My mom . . . surely loves using ellipses. She uses ellipses all the time . . . because she appreciates their function."

7.4 When you omit the end of a quoted sentence, an ellipsis follows the period. The period comes before the ellipsis and is positioned the way you would a normal period.

ORIGINAL "My mom really, truly, surely loves using ellipses, which she learned when she was nine."
EDITED "My mom really, truly, surely loves using ellipses...."
ORIGINAL "My mom said, 'I love ellipses for many reasons.'"
EDITED "My mom said, 'I love ellipses....'"

AP STYLEBOOK

AP Stylebook places a space comes between the ending period and the ellipsis.[2] *"My mom ... surely loves using ellipses. ..."*

CHICAGO

Departing from most conventional practice, *Chicago* posits that an ellipsis is **not** needed "after the last word of a quotation, even if the end of the original sentence has been omitted, unless the sentence as quoted is deliberately incomplete."[3]

ORIGINAL "My mom really, truly, surely loves using ellipses, which she learned when she was nine."
EDITED "My mom ... surely loves using ellipses."
ORIGINAL "One suitor was an incurious millionaire; the other was an engaging librarian. Choosing would be so hard, or would it be ..." [deliberately incomplete]
EDITED: "One suitor was an incurious millionaire; the other was an engaging librarian. Choosing would be so hard, or would it be ..."

7.5 If you omit the end of a quoted sentence that concludes with a period, and the sentence is followed by an in-text citation, the period comes after the in-text citation.

"And because many of us have trouble with even the simplest of marks, a proficiency in punctuation distinguishes you from the crowd ..." (citation).

7.6 If you omit the end of a quoted sentence that concludes with a question mark or exclamation point, the mark or point comes after, **not** before, the ellipsis *if* the truncated sentence still raises a question or expresses exclamation. A period follows the in-text citation, should there be one.

ORIGINAL "Aren't all these distinctions fun, assuming you define fun broadly?"
EDITED "Aren't all these distinctions fun ... ?"
EDITED "Aren't all these distinctions fun ... ?" (citation).
ORIGINAL "Knowing these distinctions is exhilarating for probably everyone!"
EDITED "Knowing these distinctions is exhilarating ... !"
EDITED "Knowing these distinctions is exhilarating ... !" (citation).

AP STYLEBOOK

Ending question marks and exclamation points come *before* the ellipsis, with a space between the ending punctuation and the ellipsis.[4] *"Aren't all these distinctions fun? ..." "Knowing these distinctions is exhilarating! ..."*

If you, the writer—**not** the quoted text—are questioning or exclaiming, the ending punctuation comes after the closing quotation mark or in-text citation.

ORIGINAL My mom, Betty Berger, said, "These distinctions are fun for a variety of reasons."
EDITED Do you agree when my mom said, "These distinctions are fun ..."?
EDITED Do you agree when my mom said, "These distinctions are fun ..." (citation)?
ORIGINAL My mom said, "These distinctions are fun for a variety of reasons."
EDITED My mom was absolutely right: "These distinctions are fun ..."!
EDITED My mom was absolutely right: "These distinctions are fun ..." (citation)!

7.7 Punctuation in the original quotation that immediately precedes or follows your insertion of an ellipsis should be maintained *if* it fits appropriately with the truncated sentence.

ORIGINAL "He was accomplished in several skills, which were hard-earned: punctuation, grammar, usage for the most part, and mechanics; the knowledge of these skills helped him to succeed in school."
EDITED "He was accomplished in several skills ...: punctuation, grammar, usage ... , and mechanics; ... these skills helped him to succeed in school."
ORIGINAL "Mark likes dogs, especially those belonging to the sporting, non-sporting, and working groups and if the dogs like rabbits; cats, if they are well-behaved, which they usually are, except for the last one he adopted; birds; horses, but only if they are Arabians, Appaloosas, and Clydesdales, and they get along with dogs, cats, and birds; rabbits; and turtles."

EDITED "Mark likes dogs, especially those belonging to the sporting, non-sporting, and working groups ... ; cats, if they are well-behaved, which they usually are ... ; birds; horses, but only if they are Arabians, Appaloosas, and Clydesdales ... ; rabbits; and turtles."

ORIGINAL "My mom really, truly, surely loves using ellipses."

EDITED "My mom really ... loves using ellipses."

7.8 If you omit one or more sentences from the original quotation, or you omit the end of one sentence along with one or more sentences that follow, represent the omission with a period and an ellipsis after the last word that comes before the omitted text. Consider this passage from William Zinsser's *On Writing Well: An Informal Guide to Writing Nonfiction*:[5]

ORIGINAL "I don't mean that some people are born clear-headed and are therefore natural writers, whereas others are naturally fuzzy and will never write well. Thinking clearly is a conscious act that the writer must force upon himself, just as if he were embarking on any other project that requires logic: adding up a laundry list or doing an algebra problem. Good writing doesn't come naturally, though most people obviously think it does. The professional writer is forever being bearded by strangers who say that they'd like to 'try a little writing some time' when they retire from their real profession. Good writing takes self-discipline, and, very often, self-knowledge."

EDITED "I don't mean that some people are born clear-headed and are therefore natural writers, whereas others are naturally fuzzy and will never write well.... Good writing doesn't come naturally.... Good writing takes self-discipline, and, very often, self-knowledge."

7.9 When you take part of one sentence and combine it with part of another, use a single ellipsis to indicate the omitted text, even if you have omitted both partial and whole sentences to form the new sentence.

ORIGINAL "A sophisticated use of punctuation will elevate your credibility with like-minded readers who value comprehensive writing skills. And because many of us have trouble with even the simplest of marks, a proficiency in punctuation distinguishes you from the crowd, increasing your worth to nearly any organization or employer."

EDITED "A sophisticated use of punctuation...distinguishes you from the crowd, increasing your worth to nearly any organization or employer."

ORIGINAL "The very process of making punctuation decisions, especially when choices present themselves, compels you to closely examine how the elements of your sentence articulate with one another with respect to which are coordinate, subordinate, and superior. Punctuation thus allows you to capture and convey the hierarchy of your thoughts."

EDITED "The very process of making punctuation decisions, especially when choices present themselves, . . . allows you to capture and convey the hierarchy of your thoughts."

CHICAGO

When quoting multiple paragraphs, *Chicago* states: "If the first part of a paragraph is omitted within a quotation, a paragraph indent and an ellipsis appear before the first quoted word. It is thus possible to use an ellipsis both at the end of one paragraph and at the beginning of the next. . . ."[6]

> This is what your quoted first paragraph would look like were you to omit text that completes the paragraph. . . .
> . . . And this is what the subsequent paragraph would look like were you to omit the beginning sentence(s).

AP STYLEBOOK

Similar to *Chicago*, *AP Stylebook* says, "When material is deleted at the end of one paragraph and at the beginning of the one that follows, place an ellipsis in both locations."[7]

> This is what your quoted first paragraph would look like were you to omit text that completes the paragraph. . . .
> . . . And this is what the subsequent paragraph would look like were you to omit the beginning sentence(s).

7.10 If you omit text that comes after a question mark or exclamation point, the mark or point takes the place of a period and is followed by an ellipsis.

ORIGINAL "Are you saying some people never use ellipses? They never, ever, use ellipses? That can't be true! I don't think so. Where did you hear such nonsense?"

EDITED "Are you saying some people never use ellipses? . . . That can't be true! . . . Where did you hear such nonsense?"

7.11 When quoting poetry, you generally observe the same ellipses guidelines that apply to prose: an ellipsis replaces any word, phrase, or sentence you omit;

if the omission comes at the end of the sentence, the ellipsis follows the closing punctuation (i.e., the period, question mark, or exclamation point). However, should you omit one or more lines from the middle of the poem, or should you omit the end of one line along with one or more lines that follow, the omission must be represented by a full line of points (periods), matching the formatted line length of the poem. If you were to abridge William Ernest Henley's "Invictus,"[8] for example, it might look something like this:

ORIGINAL Out of the night that covers me,
    Black as the pit from pole to pole,
I thank whatever gods may be
    For my unconquerable soul.

In the fell clutch of circumstance
    I have not winced nor cried aloud.
Under the bludgeonings of chance
    My head is bloody, but unbowed.

Beyond this place of wrath and tears
    Looms but the Horror of the shade,
And yet the menace of the years
    Finds and shall find me unafraid.

It matters not how strait the gate,
    How charged with punishments the scroll,
I am the master of my fate:
    I am the captain of my soul.

EDITED Out of the night that covers me,
    Black as the pit from pole to pole,
I thank whatever gods may be
    For my unconquerable soul.

In the fell clutch of circumstance
    I have not winced nor cried aloud.
. . . .
    My head is bloody, but unbowed.

. . . .
It matters not how strait the gate,
    How charged with punishments the scroll,
I am the master of my fate:
    I am the captain of my soul.

Using Ellipses as a Literary Device

7.12 Ellipses can convey theatrical pause, reflection, incomplete thought, and halting expression. Ellipses used in this way are referred to as "suspension points" because the text in some way is suspended. As Anne Toner points out in *Ellipses in English Literature: Signs of Omission*, "Ellipsis marks have developed in literary dialogue as a means of getting closer to the sounds of spoken language, to its interactivity and to the interferences that inhibit its production."[9] Suspension points find their way in fiction and informal nonfiction but rarely in academic writing. When suspension points come at the end of the sentence, **no** sentence-ending period is necessary.

- He often confused the comma with the colon as if they were in some strange way unbeknownst to everyone … *actually* alike. [theatrical pause]
- I wonder why he never learned a single rule of punctuation … [reflection]
- In the dimly lighted room, she told him that if he conquered every punctuation mark she would go out with him, let him hold her hand, and possibly … at which point he grabbed his punctuation notes, began studying, and started to imagine her …" [incomplete thought]
- I … I can't … I just can't understand why anyone would minimize the importance of punctuation. [halting expression]

7.13 If your quoted material contains an *author-generated* ellipsis, it must be labeled as such in the in-text citation (or footnote reference) that immediately follows.

> "As she looked up from her well-worn, yellow-highlighted punctuation guide, she caught the admiring gaze of a handsome gentleman holding an equally worn, yellow-highlighted copy of the same book … might this be her long-sought-after soulmate or was she just hallucinating under the pressure of learning how to use ellipses" (citation; *ellipsis in orig.*).

7.14 If you add *your* ellipsis to a text having an author-generated ellipsis, distinguish between the two. *MLA* and *Chicago* provide two options. One would be to indicate the distinction at the end of the quotation.

> "As she looked up from her well-worn, yellow-highlighted punctuation guide, she caught the admiring gaze of a handsome gentleman holding an equally worn, yellow-highlighted copy of the same book … might this be her long-sought-after soulmate or was she just hallucinating …" (citation; *1st ellipsis in orig.*).

Other possible variations for distinguishing your ellipses from those in the quoted text: (*all ellipses in orig.*), (*last ellipsis in orig.*), (*1st and 2nd ellipses in orig.*), and so forth.

A second option would be to bracket *your* ellipsis.

- "As she looked up from her well-worn, yellow-highlighted punctuation guide, she caught the admiring gaze of a handsome gentleman holding an equally worn, yellow-highlighted copy of the same book … might this be her long-sought-after soulmate or was she just hallucinating […]."

- "As she looked up from her well-worn, yellow-highlighted punctuation guide, she caught the admiring gaze of a handsome gentleman holding an equally worn, yellow-highlighted copy of the same book ... might this be her long-sought-after soulmate or was she just hallucinating [...]" (citation).

CHICAGO

When authors choose "to bracket their own ellipses," they must first explain "such a decision in a note, a preface, or elsewhere."[10]

7.15 When your quoted text ends with the *author's* ellipsis, **no** period ends the quoted text.

> "What would his parents, both English teachers, think of his dating someone who cared little about punctuation. Clearly, he was either rebelling or losing his mind. Or had he perhaps been abducted ..." (citation; *ellipsis in orig.*).

Eliminating Unnecessary Ellipses

7.16 Do **not** use ellipses to represent text that came before or after an otherwise complete quotation. If you were to quote a whole paragraph, for example, but exclude its first and last sentences, **no** ellipses would be required. Because writers seldom quote entire documents, readers can reasonably assume that additional text likely preceded and followed the quoted text.

7.17 Generally, do **not** use ellipses to indicate words omitted from the first sentence of your quoted text. Only in special contexts where exceptional precision is required, such as a legal document, must you signify changes in capitalization by bracketing the first letter of the word changed (see Chapter 6: 6.7, 6.8).

ORIGINAL The Declaration of Independence states, "We hold these truths to be self-evident, that all men are created equal, that they are endowed by their Creator with certain unalienable Rights, that among these are Life, Liberty, and the pursuit of Happiness."

INCORRECT The Declaration of Independence states, "... all men are created equal, that they are endowed by their Creator with certain unalienable Rights, that among these are Life, Liberty, and the pursuit of Happiness."

CORRECT The Declaration of Independence states, "All men are created equal, that they are endowed by their Creator with certain unalienable Rights, that among these are Life, Liberty, and the pursuit of Happiness."

7.18 Do **not** use ellipses to signify omitted material when you weave parts of the original quotation with your own text to form a seamless, coherent text.

ORIGINAL "I don't mean that some people are born clear-headed and are therefore natural writers, whereas others are naturally fuzzy and will never write well. Thinking clearly is a conscious act that the writer must force upon himself, just as if he were embarking on any other project that requires logic: adding up a laundry list or doing an algebra problem. Good writing doesn't come naturally, though most people obviously think it does. The professional writer is forever being bearded by strangers who say that they they'd like to 'try a little writing some time' when they retire from their real profession. Good writing takes self-discipline and, very often, self-knowledge."

INCORRECT William Zinsser maintains that it is not a matter of some of us being "... natural writers, whereas others are naturally fuzzy and will never write well." Rather everyone must approach writing as a "... conscious act ..." because "good writing doesn't come naturally...," but instead requires a logical approach that "... takes self-discipline and, very often, self-knowledge."

CORRECT William Zinsser maintains that it is not a matter of some of us being "natural writers, whereas others are naturally fuzzy and will never write well." Rather everyone must approach writing as "a conscious act," because "good writing doesn't come naturally," but instead requires a logical approach that "takes self-discipline and, very often, self-knowledge."

7.19 Do **not** use an ellipsis before or after a word or phrase quoted as part of single sentence.

ORIGINAL "And she also adores commas (which she always knows how to use correctly), semicolons, colons, and brackets."

INCORRECT Hazyl says that her mom "... adores ..." various punctuation marks.

CORRECT Hazyl says that her mom "adores" various punctuation marks.

ORIGINAL "My mom really, truly, surely loves using ellipses."

INCORRECT Hazyl says that her mom "... loves using ellipses."

CORRECT Hazyl says that her mom "loves using ellipses."

RHETORICALLY SPEAKING

Although it is not incorrect to use multiple ellipses when editing a quotation, a less choppy, more readable text results when you weave portions of the original quotation into your own writing. The exaggerated example below illustrates how the overuse of ellipses can hamper the flow and coherence of your text.

> William Zinsser maintains: "I don't mean that some people are ... natural writers, whereas others ... will never write well. Thinking clearly is a conscious act ... just as if [you were] ... embarking on any ... project that requires logic.... Good writing doesn't come naturally.... Good writing takes self-discipline and ... self-knowledge."

Too, the use of multiple ellipses, especially within a short span of quoted text, may appear to some readers as an attempt to massage the evidence by quoting it out of context.

More ubiquitous is the overuse of literary ellipses. Some novice writers seemingly want to end nearly every sentence with an ellipsis. Observes Toner: "The intrinsic difficulty of conveying a non-verbalized internal state is expressed typographically by the ellipsis and the common human struggle to communicate is communicated in an instant.... But its ability to be exploited as a shortcut to the meaningful brings it into disrepute and throughout its history, and not just during the twentieth century, the ellipsis oscillates as a mark of depth and banality."[11] Toner traces how various writers have long derided the excessive use of ellipses, noting that the "ellipsis is repeatedly associated with popular and often debased forms of writing. It is as much a sin as a sign of omission. The ellipsis is a form of mechanical mood-setting, an evasion adopted by the hasty and inadequate author or a genre-based cliché."[12]

ELLIPSIS: KEY DIFFERENCES BETWEEN AMERICAN AND BRITISH STYLE

❖ *Oxford Style* includes a space before and after the ellipsis but **no** spaces between the points of the ellipsis.[13] (Quotations below have been placed in single quotation marks to reflect British style.)

'My mom ... surely loves using ellipses.'

❖ When a period (or question mark or exclamation point) comes before an ellipsis, a space is usually left between the ending punctuation and the ellipsis.[14]

'I don't mean that some people are born clear-headed and are therefore natural writers, whereas others are naturally fuzzy and will never write well. ... Good writing doesn't come naturally. ... Good writing takes self-discipline, and, very often, self-knowledge.'

> ❖ British style, similar to American style, includes **no** sentence-ending period when suspension points come at the end of a sentence.[15] "When an incomplete sentence is an embedded quotation within a larger complete sentence," however, "the normal sentence full point is added after the final quotation mark."[16]
>
> She would often wander the hallways, mumbling to herself, 'I wonder why he never learned a single rule of punctuation ...'.

Slashes

Pairing Words

7.20 Use a slash to indicate choice (between one or the other) in paired words, as in *yes/no*, *he/she*, *pass/fail*, *win/lose*. In these cases, the slash (with **no** space before or after) replaces the word *or*.

7.21 Use a slash to unite paired words, as in *owner/operator*, *writer/director*, *player/coach*, *washer/dryer*, *May/June issue*. In these cases, the slash (with **no** space before or after) replaces the word *and*.

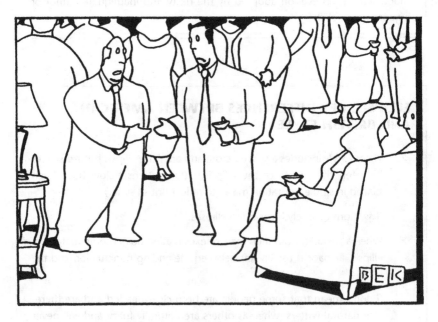

"I'm a wunderkind slash flop."

Bruce Eric Kaplan/The New Yorker Collection/The Cartoon Bank; Condé Nast

CHICAGO

Chicago suggests, "Where one or more of the terms separated by slashes is an open compound [two or more words that combine to produce a new, single meaning], a space before and after the slash can make the text more legible."[17] For example:

> wealth manager / financial planner

Such holds true for hyphenated compounds as well, such as:

> mother-in-law / father-in-law

When the space is reduced between the two compounds, they are a bit less legible, as seen here:

* wealth manager/financial planner
* mother-in-law/father-in-law

RHETORICALLY SPEAKING

By replacing *or* and *and*, words that implicitly rank their preceding and following text, the slash more democratically unites the paired items and better establishes each as equal. However, the meaning—and power—of the slash is compromised when it is unclear whether it replaces *or* or *and*. In *teacher/ scholar*, for example, is the intended meaning *teacher or scholar* or *teacher and scholar*?). Moreover, sometimes the slash simultaneously speaks to both choice and combination. *And/or*, for example, provides the reader with two possible readings. *You will be tested next Monday and/or Tuesday on how to use a slash* could mean either of the following:

* You will be tested next Monday or Tuesday on how to use a slash.
  Or:
* You will be tested next Monday and Tuesday on how to use a slash.

Fowler cautions, "*And/or* linking more than two items is to be avoided at all costs: *Social variation in language may be due to social class, ethnic origin, age, and/or sex* leaves it bafflingly unclear with which other facts 'sex' is associated."[18] Such potential ambiguity explains why the slash is less favored in formal writing, where greater precision is expected.

Still, the slash enables you to avoid bulky constructions that can appear in complex sentence structures. If you were to differentiate between a writer's main ideas and main arguments and then speak of them and their sub-structure collectively, you might say, *The author's main ideas/main arguments and her subideas/subarguments consistently address* ... Here the use of slashes makes the sentence easier to read than if you were to write, *The author's main ideas and main arguments and her subideas and subarguments consistently address* ...

Sometimes the slash can even enhance clarity. *You should preview what you are about to describe/explain or argue* speaks of two options. *You should preview what you are about to describe or explain or argue* suggests three.

Separating Lines of Poetry

7.22 Use a slash (with a space before and after the slash) to separate lines of quoted poetry when they are short enough to be included in your text, rather than separated into a block quotation.

In her poem, "A Word Is Dead," Emily Dickinson contrasts one view of language—"A word is dead/When it is said,/Some say"—to that of her own: "I say it just/Begins to live/That day."[19]

Abbreviating and Formatting Information

7.23 Use a slash in informal abbreviations of dates (12/25/89; 2010/11) and certain words and phrases (A/C; c/o; $45/oz.); and in formatting URL addresses (www.routledge.com/cw/kallan) and numerical fractions (3/4; 9½).

Notes

1 *AP Stylebook*, 324.
2 *AP Stylebook*, 325.
3 *Chicago*, 729.
4 *AP Stylebook*, 325.
5 William Zinsser, *On Writing Well: An Informal Guide to Writing Nonfiction* (New York: Harper & Row, 1976), 9.
6 *Chicago*, 730–31.
7 *AP Stylebook*, 325.
8 William Ernest Henley, *A Book of Verses* (London: David Nutt in the Strand, 1888), 56–57.
9 Anne Toner, *Ellipses in English Literature: Signs of Omission* (Cambridge: Cambridge University Press, 2015), 5.
10 *Chicago*, 732.
11 Toner, 13.

12 Toner, 3.
13 *Oxford Style*, 81–82.
14 *Oxford Style*, 82.
15 *Oxford Style*, 82.
16 *Oxford Style*, 82.
17 *Chicago*, 405.
18 Butterfield, ed., *Fowler's Dictionary*, 50.
19 *The Poems of Emily Dickinson*, ed. Thomas H. Johnson, 845.

8

PARENTHESES AND BRACKETS

Purpose and Application

Parentheses ( ) and brackets [ ] enclose information incidental or less relevant to your main point; only the explanatory footnote is more incidental.[1] Parentheses and brackets usually signal the presentation of detail worthy enough to include, but **not** important enough to grammatically integrate with the rest of the sentence.

Parentheses and brackets serve other functions as well. By allowing the writer to distinctly label material as incidental, parentheses announce the writer's focus and direct the reader's attention appropriately. Parentheses and brackets in the context of quoted material clearly stipulate whether it is the writer or the quoted source who is speaking. And the use of brackets in bibliographic entries can effectively separate data to enhance legibility.

Parentheses

Subordinating Information

8.1 Use parentheses to subordinate less important information, allowing for a more coherent, more focused message. In the two passages below, notice how the second benefits from parentheses.

- Parentheses can be a helpful writing tool. The singular of *parentheses* is *parenthesis*. However, parentheses should not be overused. Parentheses are my grandmother's favorite form of punctuation.
- Parentheses (singular, *parenthesis*) can be a helpful writing tool. However, parentheses (my grandmother's favorite form of punctuation) should not be overused.

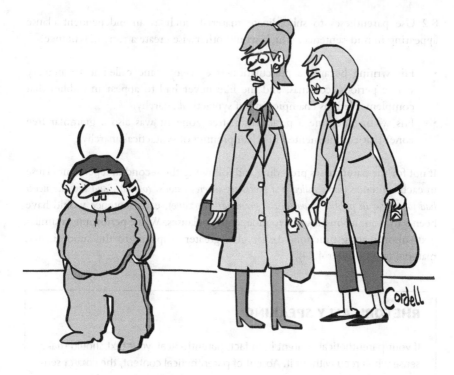

"I blame the parentheses."

Cordell, Tim; www.CartoonStock.com

In the example above, parenthetical information takes the form of explanation and editorial digression, both of which, while **not** crucial to the functioning of the sentence, can be helpful and interesting to the reader. Here are more examples of how parenthetical comment can add value to your text:

- Parentheses (from the Greek word *parentithenai*, meaning to put aside) should not be confused with brackets.
- In Great Britain (England, Scotland, and Wales), brackets are called *square brackets*, and parentheses are referred to as *round brackets*.
- Many of my college friends (notably Don, Ed, and Bob) do not care as much about parentheses as I do.
- Most members of the National Council of Teachers of English (NCTE) know a thing or two about parentheses.
- My last girlfriend (I broke up with her after four weeks) was definitely parentheses challenged.

8.2 Use parentheses to subordinate material, such as an independent clause appearing in mid-sentence, which would otherwise create a run-on sentence.

- His writing became a punctuation-free zone (some called it a sanctuary where periods, commas, and the like never had to appear in public) that complemented his championing of syntactical anarchy.
- His writing became a punctuation-free zone (it was also a grammar-free zone) that complemented his championing of syntactical anarchy.

If not for the parentheses preceding and following the second independent clause in each sentence (*some called it a sanctuary where periods, commas, and the like never had to appear in public*; *it was also a grammar-free zone*), each sentence would have been a run-on, having fused two independent clauses. While performing a similar text-subordinating function, dashes give greater emphasis to the subordinated material (see Chapter 4.14).

RHETORICALLY SPEAKING

If your parenthetical content is, in fact, parenthetical, your text should make sense when read without it. Absent of parenthetical content, the CORRECT sentence in the following two examples grammatically coheres; the INCORRECT sentence does not.

INCORRECT Although they easily learned (for example, how to use periods, question marks, and exclamation points), mastering the intricacies of the comma proved more challenging.

CORRECT Although they easily learned how to use ending punctuation (for example, periods, question marks, and exclamation points), mastering the intricacies of the comma proved more challenging.

INCORRECT Punctuation (and, of course, grammar) are my favorite subjects.

CORRECT Punctuation (and, of course, grammar) is my favorite subject.

These examples treat parenthetical material as separate from the sentence's grammatical structure. A contrary view is offered by Dryer: "An 'and' is an 'and,' and the use of parentheses (or commas or dashes) to break up a plural subject for whatever reason does not negate the pluralness of the subject." Dryer would thus write: *Punctuation (and, of course, grammar) are my favorite subjects.* But, he adds, if the parenthetical comment had begun with "to say nothing of" or "not to mention," the subject would be singular: *Punctuation (to say nothing of grammar) is important to know.*[2]

Positioning Commas with Parentheses

8.3 Do **not** place a comma before a beginning parenthesis or before an ending parenthesis.

INCORRECT Although they easily learned how to use ending punctuation, (periods, question marks, and exclamation points) mastering the intricacies of the comma proved more challenging.

INCORRECT Although they easily learned how to use ending punctuation (periods, question marks, and exclamation points,) mastering the intricacies of the comma proved more challenging.

CORRECT Although they easily learned how to use ending punctuation (periods, question marks, and exclamation points), mastering the intricacies of the comma proved more challenging.

INCORRECT They owned cars that were German, (two Volkswagens) British, (three Jaguars) Italian, (a Ferrari) and Japanese (four Toyotas).

INCORRECT They owned cars that were German (two Volkswagens,) British (three Jaguars,) Italian (a Ferrari,) and Japanese (four Toyotas).

CORRECT They owned cars that were German (two Volkswagens), British (three Jaguars), Italian (a Ferrari), and Japanese (four Toyotas).

Enclosing Numbers and Letters with Parentheses

8.4 Use parentheses to enclose numbers or letters that serve to label items appearing within the body of a paragraph. Avoid using a single parenthesis, which, as will now be demonstrated, 1) only partially encloses/separates the letter or number from its preceding and following text and 2) appears incomplete. A paired parenthesis (which marks a beginning and an end), on the other hand, (1) fully encloses/separates the text, thereby creating more legibility, and (2) appears more balanced and complete.

Note: **No** period follows a number or letter enclosed by parentheses (see Chapter 1: 1.11).

Eliminating Unnecessary Parentheses

8.5 Do **not** use parentheses for enclosing numbers or letters that are vertically formatted. Periods alone provide sufficient visual separation between the number or letter and the text that follows (see Chapter 1: 1.2).

Three steps must be taken:
1. text ...   A. text ...
2. text ...   B. text ...
3. text ...   C. text ...

(See Chapter 1 for how to position periods, question marks, and exclamation points with parentheses.)

8.6 Do **not** place parentheses within parentheses (nested parentheses) in a narrative text.

INCORRECT My last boyfriend, Billy Android Duke (yes, his initials spelled BAD (can you believe it?) and he put his initials on everything) was parentheses challenged.

Instead, place the second parentheses in brackets (see 8.9) or, better yet, revise the sentence.

CORRECT My last boyfriend, Billy Android Duke (yes, his initials spelled BAD— can you believe it?—and he put his initials on everything) was parentheses challenged.
CORRECT My last boyfriend, Billy Android Duke (can you believe his initials spelled BAD and that he would sign everything with those initials?) was definitely parentheses challenged.

Note: Some style manuals allow for parentheses within parentheses when compiling bibliographic entries. The practice, for example, is common in legal documents.

> The District Court denied Citizens United's motion for a preliminary injunction, 530 F. Supp. 2d 274 (D.D.C. 2008) (per curiam), and then granted the FEC's motion for summary judgment, App. 261a–262a. See id., at 261a ("Based on the reasoning of our prior opinion, we find that the [FEC] is entitled to judgment as a matter of law. See Citizen[s] United v. FEC, 530 F. Supp. 2d 274 (D.D.C. 2008) (denying Citizens United's request for a preliminary injunction)").[3]

RHETORICALLY SPEAKING

Parenthetical asides are sometimes used in informal texts as a way of humanizing the writer by revealing one's inner—and seemingly earnest— thoughts.

> I have no idea (like absolutely *no* idea) why the professor asked me to consider rewriting my paper (and it *really* was my paper in case you were wondering) for publication.

Brackets

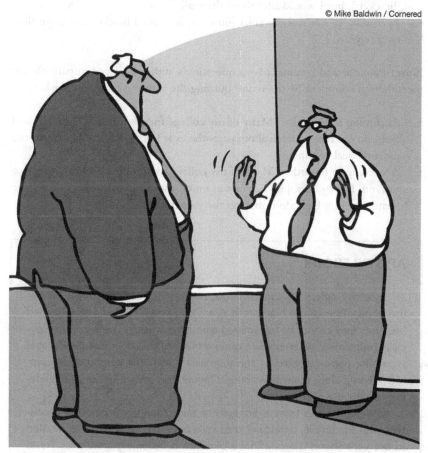

© Mike Baldwin / Cornered

"I'll stop using finger quotes if you
(control freak) let me use hand brackets."

Baldwin, Mike; www.CartoonStock.com

Commenting Editorially

8.7 When you need or want to editorially comment within the body of a quotation, place your words in brackets, **not** in parentheses. Bracketed commentary
allows you to offer immediate explanation, clarification, and perspective about
the original quotation.

- His autobiography began unusually: "While at Oxford, I learned how to use
  round brackets [also known as parentheses]."

- "They [his classmates at Oxford] thought I did not know how to use them [brackets], but I would later show them all."
- According to her dad, "Ivanka [now 19] has loved brackets for more than twenty years."

Note: Parenthetical comment by a quotation's author is placed in parentheses; parenthetical comment by the writer quoting the author is placed in brackets.

- According to Ricardo, "Many of my college friends (notably Don, Ed, and Bob) do not care as much about parentheses as I do." [Ricardo is making the parenthetical comment.]
- According to Ricardo, "Many of my college friends [he's probably referring to Don, Ed, and Bob] do not care as much about parentheses as I do." [The writer quoting Ricardo is making the parenthetical comment.]

AP STYLEBOOK

AP Stylebook differs significantly from other style manuals relative to the use of parentheses and brackets. It states that brackets should **not** be used because "they cannot be transmitted over news wires."[4] This becomes especially problematic when reading quoted material that does **not** clearly label who—the person quoted or the journalist—owns the parenthetical comment. Fortunately, many news outlets follow their own in-house style guidelines on the use of brackets.

AP Stylebook also takes a dim view of parentheses, a perspective consistent with the simple, unencumbered style of newswriting: "The temptation to use parentheses is a clue that a sentence is becoming contorted. Try to write it another way. If a sentence must contain incidental material, then commas or two dashes are frequently more effective."[5]

8.8 Use brackets to let your reader know that an obvious error in the quotation was committed by the author, **not** you. *The editor wrote that I needed to fix "all the instances where you're* [sic] *use of contractions is incorrect."* Lest you appear petty, however, use *sic* selectively to acknowledge only the most striking of errors or nonstandard spellings that would likely draw the reader's attention.

Bracketing Parenthetical Information within Parentheses

8.9 Parenthetical information that appears *within* a text enclosed by parentheses should be bracketed. Most often, this occurs in bibliographic entries.

- "Nearly 70% of all college students misuse brackets (*Journal of Bracket Research* 24.7 [2018]: 63)."
- Some may live a happier life if they master parentheses and brackets (see Myrwin [2017, 2019], whose longitudinal studies of punctuation link correct bracket use with financial success).

An exception—parentheses appearing within brackets—can be found in mathematical equations and chemical formulas, where parentheses aid in legibility by separating data that would otherwise run together. Additionally, parentheses in mathematical equations specify the order of calculations.

$$[(8 + 4) \times (4 - 2) - 6] \times 2 = [(6 - 3) \times (1 + 2) \times 4] = 36$$

Nickel Carbonyl $[Ni(CO)_4]$ \qquad Iron Carbonyl $[Fe(CO)_5]$

Editing Quotations

8.10 When you shorten or grammatically revise a quotation to fit your purposes, use bracketed wording to ensure your edited text is coherent.

ORIGINAL "A paper graded in pencil connotes a less foreboding instructor whose comments and suggestions seem more advisory than absolute. Easy on the ego, the penciled critique is most fitting when reviewing the work of colleagues with whom you want to remain friends."

ADAPTATION "A paper graded in pencil...seem[s] more advisory than absolute ... [and] is most fitting when reviewing the work of colleagues with whom you want to remain friends."

RHETORICALLY SPEAKING

It is tempting to offer parenthetical and bracketed comment in academic writing, which favors detail, nuance, and qualification. But reading a text with multiple parenthetical and bracketed asides often proves taxing, each aside interrupting the flow of the sentence and potentially impeding its readability. Parentheses and brackets should be used sparingly, and, in some cases, not at all if the comment can be set off more effectively by other means.

In the example below, the parenthetical material in the ORIGINAL would function better if it were enclosed by commas because it is more central to the sentence's purpose and thus deserving of greater integration and emphasis within the sentence.

ORIGINAL When asked about today's music, Moses (92), said he thought that hip-hop was not music and that his musical hero (Al Jolson) would have agreed.

REVISED When asked about today's music, Moses, 92, said he thought that hip-hop was not music and that his musical hero, Al Jolson, would have agreed.

When a parenthetical comment warrants greater emphasis than normally afforded by parentheses (or even commas), dashes prove more appropriate. The revised version below, compared to the original, better highlights the point of the sentence.

ORIGINAL Moses said he disliked (no, he actually *hated*) today's music.
REVISED Moses said he disliked—no, he actually *hated*—today's music.

In other cases, the parenthetical comment, owing to its length or its lack of contextual significance, can bog down the message, distracting the reader from a more fluid, unimpeded reading of the text. Such parenthetical comment may be better expressed as an explanatory footnote.

PARENTHESES AND BRACKETS: KEY DIFFERENCES BETWEEN AMERICAN AND BRITISH STYLE

❖ Parentheses are referred to as *round brackets*, and brackets are called *square brackets*.[6]

❖ *Oxford Style* advises to generally avoid nested parentheses, but concedes: "This is sometimes inevitable, as when matter mentioned parenthetically already contains parentheses. In such cases Oxford prefers double parentheses to square brackets within parentheses (the usual US convention)."[7] *I broke up with my boyfriend, Billy Android Duke (yes, his initials spelled BAD (can you believe it?)).*

Notes

1 Technically, a *parenthesis* comprises a single curved mark) or a pair of curved marks ( ). *Parentheses*, however, is commonly used to refer to a pair, as well as pairs, of curved marks.
2 Dryer, *Dryer's English*, 46.
3 Citizens United v. Federal Election Commission, 558 U.S. 310, 322 (2010).
4 *AP Stylebook*, 321–22.
5 *AP Stylebook*, 326–27.
6 *Oxford Style*, 88.
7 *Oxford Style*, 90.

INDEX

Printed in the United States
by Baker & Taylor Publisher Services

Printed in the United States
by Baker & Taylor Publisher Services